Consent Practices in Performing Arts Education

Consent Practices in Performing Arts Education

Elaine DiFalco Daugherty and
Heather Trommer-Beardslee

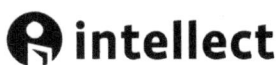

ᗺ intellect

Bristol, UK / Chicago, USA

First published in the UK in 2024 by
Intellect, The Mill, Parnall Road, Fishponds, Bristol, BS16 3JG, UK

First published in the USA in 2024 by
Intellect, The University of Chicago Press, 1427 E. 60th Street,
Chicago, IL 60637, USA

A catalogue record for this book is available from
the British Library.

Copy editor: MPS Limited
Cover designer: Tanya Montefusco
Cover image: Michael Armistead
Production manager: Julie Willis (Westchester Publishing Services UK)
Typesetter: MPS Limited

Hardback print ISBN 978-1-78938-971-5
Paperback print ISBN 978-1-78938-973-9
ePDF ISBN 978-1-78938-972-2
ePUB ISBN 978-1-78938-970-8

To find out about all our publications, please visit our website.
There you can subscribe to our e-newsletter, browse or download our current
catalogue and buy any titles that are in print.

www.intellectbooks.com

This is a peer-reviewed publication.

Contents

Figures

Acknowledgments

A substantial element of our research included conducting a series of interviews with people of varying professions including comedy, music, theatre and dance educators, consent educators, intimacy organization founders, professional performers and directors, and a Title IX coordinator. The following is a list of the people who generously shared their time with us.

Patsy Collins Bandes
Carly DW Bones
Brandon Chu
Kimberley Cooper
Jamie Freeman Cormack
Dan Daugherty
Rachel Finley
Deborah Hertzberg
Ann James
Brian Kremer
LaToya Lain
Sarah Lozoff
Andreé Martin
Betty Martin
Mary Martinez
Joshua May

Chels Morgan
Chelsea Pace
Nicole Perry
Kelly Quinnett
Ashley Reade
Laura Rikard
Liz Joynt Sandberg
Mia Schachter
Keeley Stanley-Bohn
Jessica Steinrock
Zev Steinrock
Claire-Frances Sullivan
Daniel Thieme-Whitlow
Tommy Wedge
Stephan Wilson

Introduction

As performing arts educators, our responsibility to our students requires that we not only train them, but that we keep our training current with the industry standards. Setting students up for career longevity necessitates preparation for the rigorous physical and emotional tolls the work may take on them. It also means providing any available tools to mitigate those tolls. This includes teaching and modeling consent practices that value and prioritize body autonomy. Instituting these practices not only provides a productive learning experience for our current students but also allows us to send practitioners into their professional careers with these values firmly in place and with expectations set for how to treat and be treated by others. Eventually, these values and expectations permeate the performing arts industries and become the new standard. Consent-based praxis, which has been around in conversation and action outside of the realm of the performing arts for a very long time, must infiltrate all of our interactions with our students and the cultures we create in each learning environment.

Many of us who have worked in the performing arts for a long time have heard the following phrases, or something eerily similar, time and time again:

"This is how I teach because this is how I was taught."

"It was uncomfortable, but my director told me to, so I did it."

"I wanted the job, so I did what I was told."

In fact, we, Elaine DiFalco Daugherty (theatre professor) and Heather Trommer-Beardslee (dance professor) have said those things ourselves—especially as it relates to practices in the classroom involving touch as a teaching, directing, or choreographic tool. We have touched students without consent as we were teaching and making physical corrections in movement classes. We have had students touch each other in the context of shows and rehearsals without first engaging in boundary conversations designed to create open lines of communication and clear expectations for individual wellness. As we are writing this, it is worth noting that we are cringing, because seeing these words in print looks really alarming. When we reflect on past behaviors from a time when we were less equipped with knowledge and tools, it can elicit feelings of shame. And yet, we taught the way we were taught, we directed the way we were directed. This is not an excuse by any means, but an acknowledgment of shared histories and the growing desire for change that creates learning environments in which everyone values their autonomy and the autonomy of others. During our interview with Zev Steinrock, assistant professor of Acting and Stage Combat at the University of Illinois, Urbana—Champaign, he reminded us, "To be part of this change in the performing arts industry, you have to be comfortable with looking back at your prior practices over and over and over again and learn to not implode with shame" (Steinrock 2022). Shame can be destructive and not a helpful part in making real, productive change. Creating consent-forward spaces means moving on and moving ahead.

In 2018, Elaine attended a panel at the Association for Theatre in Higher Education Annual Conference with Theatrical Intimacy Education (TIE) (Busselle et al. 2018), a relatively new organization focused on the very-new-at-the-time specialization of intimacy direction. When it was done, she walked across the hall for her next session and participated in a choreography workshop (Pace and DuVal 2018) with them. It turns out that this was the beginning of a journey that would lead to countless hours of training in workshops with TIE, Intimacy Directors International (IDI), Intimacy Directors and Coordinators (IDC), Heartland Intimacy Design and Training, as well as training in diversity, equity, and inclusion, bystander intervention, mental health first aid, and additional supplemental areas of interest.

This training led to a thesis project for her MFA work at the University of Idaho focused on intimacy direction and consent practices (Daugherty 2020). Since it was a distance program, Elaine worked with her students at Central Michigan University (CMU) on her projects involving consent-forward practices and the development of her pedagogy. Unequivocally, they were excited about this work. In many ways, they were shocked to learn that they actually have control over their own bodies when it comes to classroom and production-based learning. Why is this shocking news to students? Well, because in many ways, we as educators and performance practitioners ourselves have perpetuated the problem by not stating our own boundaries and in turn have created learning environments that aren't actually rooted in a culture of consent-forward practices. Sarah Lozoff, intimacy director for American Ballet Theatre and RudduR Dance, explains her experience working with professional dancers,

> I have never seen such control over one's own body—all of their limbs—all of their extremities—control over every movement. Yet by and large, what I've witnessed is

that this group of performers feels the least amount of agency over their own bodies. That is a very hard dichotomy.

(Lozoff 2022)

We witnessed the very same thing in terms of a perceived lack of agency with our university dance and theatre students.

With Elaine's investigation, something was brewing at CMU. The conversation started and it soon erupted into an unstoppable force of students interested in learning more about this practice of consent-based performance education and creation. The movement became contagious at CMU and Heather began asking about how the foundational consent practices of intimacy design could be translated to dance classrooms and rehearsal spaces. In other words, how do we create consent-to-touch practices for the dance studio as an alternative to assuming that every student is okay with being touched because they showed up in the class-room or in the rehearsal space? As we considered this translation of practices, our inquiry expanded to focus on performing arts education in a broader scope in order to apply consent theory to a wider base of educational environments. As we set out on this research journey, we asked ourselves the following questions:

How is consent being defined? How do we define consent in the context of performing arts education?

What is happening in higher education performing arts classrooms to engage in consent practices? What are educators doing? How are they doing it? How is it going?

What do we need to be doing as educators to model consent-forward behaviors?

Methodology (How We Sought Answers to Our Questions)

We read (a lot). The breadth of our sources was broad. We read about consent and its varied definitions across and between disparate fields of study. We read about how the topic of consent is addressed by Title IX for college campuses across the country. We read about power and power dynamics, the effects of the COVID-19 pandemic on our collective mental and emotional well-being, and the ways inti-macy and consent educators are breaking down historically impervious walls to make way for greater empathy, gratitude, and safety in our educational spaces.

Mostly, however, we listened and digested. We administered an IRB-approved survey about the use of touch in performing arts classrooms. We conducted dozens of interviews with people of varying professions including comedy, music, theatre

3

and dance educators, consent educators, intimacy organization founders, professional performers and directors, and a Title IX coordinator. These narratives were essential to our understanding of what is currently being done and peoples' goals for the future ... the what's next in the consent-based performing arts education world. The people we interviewed ranged from experts in the field of intimacy direction with robust, curated consent practices to some educators who are just starting to contemplate implementing some of these consent-forward practices into their own classrooms and rehearsal spaces. Many were implementing consent-based practices without implicitly having conversations about these practices with their students. The interviews from all across the implementation spectrum, from beginning stages to experts in the field, were equally valuable. We found that each person opened up a new window of understanding in this multi-layered complexity of educational theory and practice work that is human-centric at its core. It's important to note that after the interviews and initial writing process, we sent each cited interviewee the writing that referenced them and the context in which it was going to live. We offered each contributor options to edit or veto material to be included. We view this practice as another act of consent and are telling you, the reader, of this so that you know that the intimate ideas and stories that are shared in this book, are done so with permission granted through our own active consent practices.

A Selection of Notable Organizations, Scholarship, and Interview Highlights

Conversations surrounding consent are certainly not new. While its codified place in theatre is a fairly recent development, conversations about consent as it relates to bodily autonomy have been taking place for a long time. Significant contributors to the field of consent education include, but are not limited to, The Consent Academy, Consent Wizardry, Betty Martin, Cuddle Party, Creating Consent Culture, Intimacy Coordinators of Color, Intimacy Directors and Coordinators, Theatrical Intimacy Education, Momentum Stage, National Society of Intimacy Professionals, Principal Intimacy Professionals, and Intimacy for Stage and Screen. Some of these organizations are strictly focused on consent education while others are organizations with consent at the center of their artistic work. In her book, *Staging Sex: Best Practices, Tools, and Techniques for Theatrical Intimacy*, Chelsea Pace writes, "It's not enough to tell actors they can say 'no.' We need to normalize 'no' and we do that by establishing an expectation, with words and with our actions, that everyone will have boundaries and those boundaries will be respected" (2020: 10). In The Chicago Theatre Standards and Not In Our House online living document, the following is stated,

When creative environments are unsafe, both the artist and the art can become compromised. Spaces that prize "raw," "violent," and otherwise high—risk material can veer into unsafe territory if there are no procedures for prevention, communication, and when necessary, response.

(Not In Our House December 2017)

It is our goal as authors, educators, and performance practitioners to have open conversations about consent and boundary protection as they relate to varying learning structures. This takes focused work to engage in teaching and performance creation methods that open up the possibilities for all learners. Our students don't arrive with uniform experiences, histories, backgrounds, identities, or cultures. Consent-forward work is part of our opportunity as educators to create clearer pathways to learning within educational structures for a more diverse student body.

Though colleges are more diverse than in previous generations, race continues to matter in how students view these environments. Moreover, racial identity intersects with other identities and positions that students hold. In turn, negative and positive perceptions influence student experiences and outcomes. Cultivating postsecondary environments where all students, regardless of racial background, pathway into college, and other social identities, feel supported requires intentional action.

(Cuellar and Johnson-Ahorlu 2019: 41)

In addition to this vital need for intentional action, Ann James, the founding director of Intimacy Coordinators of Color, spoke about the power of narrative and historical connection to the present.

We are here because of our ancestors. I am somatically aligned with the DNA of my ancestors running through my veins. I am guided by their undeniable wisdom to survive on a day-to-day basis and this brings clarity to my understanding of consent and respect for all people in a shared room.

(James 2022)

These contemplations and assertions were pivotal for us as we navigated our own understanding(s), memories, and relationships with educational practices that are truly human centered and the complications entrenched in such dynamics.

How This All Works Together

The move toward integrating consent practices more succinctly into the performing arts may have emerged with the intimacy movement, but implementing consent practices can't only be the work of intimacy specialists; it has to be everyone's responsibility. This book expands the discussion of consent as a foundational tenet of intimacy direction by focusing on creating and sustaining a culture of active consent in higher education classrooms and rehearsal spaces across the performing arts. It covers consent as a foundational element in undergraduate performance education and how to apply that in the rehearsal space as classroom lessons are applied to more fully produced performance projects. Each chapter was written with the understanding that the information will need to be adapted to fit a wide variety of performing arts classrooms in terms of genres and teaching capacities. With this in mind, a variety of examples and suggestions are included in order to meet varying needs.

Chapter 1 defines and outlines the foundational principles of consent and power dynamics and connects this discussion to performing arts classrooms and production spaces. Chapter 2 includes our IRB-approved survey results, details the philosophies behind creating programmatic consent policies, and provides examples for getting started. Chapter 3 outlines methods of modeling consent-forward behavior in the classroom, establishing and fostering an environment that values autonomy and agency, and non-touch and/or low-touch teaching techniques. Sample syllabus language is included that may be used in setting up classroom expectations. Chapter 4 is a continuation of the content discussed in Chapter 3 and translates the information to the production space. Chapter 5 includes activities and strategies designed to help students embrace their autonomy. It is a collection generously provided for inclusion in this book by practitioners currently working in the performing arts. Chapter 6 provides real-life examples of how consent is informing individual or departmental teaching practices in performing arts classrooms and the learning lessons that have shaped our histories. The Conclusion includes a message about the impossibility of perfection, the highlights, and quick tips for getting started.

During our interview with LaToya Lain, assistant professor of music at the University of North Carolina—Chapel Hill, she explained,

> We need to grow accustomed to initiating, modeling, and encouraging conversations about consent. Until this practice becomes the norm, student-teacher dynamics will continue to feel awkward and uncomfortable. Most students desire this conversation. They are leaning into the idea that they have authority over their own bodies and their own spaces.
>
> (Lain 2022)

This book is a way for us, as educators, to do just that. It is not our intention to define the "right way" to create a consent-forward classroom because we don't believe there is one right way to do it. There is an expanse of ideas and perspectives that can be brought to this work which influences how it shows up in our spaces. We have included options and ideas that we hope may guide you on a journey of discovering methods that are best suited to your students' needs and yours.

In our interview with Laura Rikard, co-founder and head faculty of Theatrical Intimacy Education and assistant professor of Theatre at the University of South Carolina Upstate, she explained,

> I think of it as a baker who makes the best wedding cakes and is now questioning why they need to include these new ingredients. I respond by saying "I respect that you know how to do what you do and I am not telling you that you have to change everything that you do. This is an offering and I can provide you with evidence of how it will make things better for people in the space, but I am only going to ask if you can start with one of these tools and you can see where it goes from there."
>
> (Rikard 2022)

Following Laura's lead, this book is just that ... an offering. It is a collection of ideas, exercises, and personal narratives that may be a useful companion on your teaching journey. This book was crafted with care as a model for the embodied intentions we hope to pass on to those who enter our classrooms and production spaces.

REFERENCES

Busselle, K., Pace, C., Rikard, L., Shawyer, S. and Shively, K. (2018), "Best practices for intimacy and violence on stage," *Association for Theatre in Higher Education Annual Conference*, Boston, MA, Thursday, 2 August.

Consent Wizardry (n.d.), https://consentwizardry.com. Accessed 19 August 2023.

Creating Consent Culture (n.d.), https://www.creatingconsentculture.com. Accessed 19 August 2023.

Cuddle Party (n.d.), https://cuddleparty.com. Accessed 19 August 2023.

Cuellar, Marcela G. and Johnson-Ahorlu, R. Nicole (2019), "The contingent climate: Exploring student perspectives at a racially diverse institution," in C. W. Byrd, R. J. Brunn-Bevel and S. M. Ovink (eds), *Intersectionality and Higher Education*, New Brunswick, NJ: Rutgers University Press, p. 41.

Daugherty, E. D. (2020), "Intimacy direction: Emerging pedagogy in practice," unpublished master's thesis, Moscow, ID: University of Idaho.

Heartland Intimacy Design and Training (n.d.), https://www.heartlandintimacydesign.com. Accessed 19 August 2023.

Intimacy Coordinators of Color (n.d.), https://www.intimacycoordinatorsofcolor.com. Accessed 19 August 2023.

Intimacy Directors and Coordinators (n.d.), https://idcprofessionals.com. Accessed 19 August 2023.

Intimacy Directors and Coordinators (n.d.), "IDC is a new company formed by many of the intimacy professionals who were heavily involved at IDI: IDI has been dissolved as of March 2020," https://idcprofessionals.com/faqs. Accessed 15 July 2023.

Intimacy for Stage and Screen (n.d.), https://www.intimacyforstageandscreen.com. Accessed 19 August 2023.

James, A. (2022), interviewed by E. Daugherty and H. Trommer-Beardslee, Online 24 May 2022.

Lain, L. (2022), interviewed by E. Daugherty and H. Trommer-Beardslee, Online 14 June 2022.

Lozoff, S. (2022), interviewed by E. Daugherty and H. Trommer-Beardslee, Online 1 June 2022.

Martin, Betty (n.d.), https://bettymartin.org. Accessed 19 August 2023.

Momentum Stage (n.d.), https://www.momentumstage.org. Accessed 19 August 2023.

National Society of Intimacy Professionals (n.d.), https://intimacysociety.com. Accessed 19 August 2023.

Not In Our House (2017), "#NotInOurHouse: A Chicago Theatre Community," https://www.notinourhouse.org/. Accessed 29 August 2022.

Pace, C. and DuVal, C. (2018), "Playing it safe: A foundational fight and intimacy choreography workshop for acting and directing teachers," *Association for Theatre in Higher Education Annual Conference*, Boston, MA, 2 August.

Pace, C. and Rikard, L. (2020), *Staging Sex: Best Practices, Tools, and Techniques for Theatrical Intimacy*, London: Routledge, p. 10.

Principal Intimacy Professionals (n.d.), https://www.principalintimacy.com. Accessed 19 August 2023.

Rikard, L. (2022), interviewed by E. Daugherty and H. Trommer-Beardslee, Online 14 May 2022.

Steinrock, Z. (2022), interviewed by E. Daugherty and H. Trommer-Beardslee, Online 26 May 2022.

Theatrical Intimacy Education (n.d.), https://www.theatricalintimacyed.com. Accessed 19 August 2023.

The Consent Academy (n.d.), https://www.consent.academy/. Accessed 19 August 2023.

1

Consent and Power Dynamics

Consent

The semantics and ideologies surrounding consent are complicated. The practice of consent looks and sounds different from situation to situation and from person to person.

> Consent informs every movement in the dance between individual autonomy and relationship with others. What at first glance appears to be a simple matter of yes or no becomes a complex web of unconscious expectations, self-esteem, societal status, unexamined beliefs, systemic manipulation, and more.
> (Baczynski and Scott 2022: 31)

It is a difficult subject to quantify because it inherently exists within a myriad of interrelated conditions. There are any number of variations of definitions for consent, the specifics of which can change based on the particular framework of the experience to which it applies. A legal definition of consent vs. a medical definition of informed consent vs. Title IX's definition of consent—they are all variations on a similar idea, but not so much so that they could be swapped out one for another.

Typically, if people are engaged in discussions about consent, it is primarily focused on navigating consent as a means to navigating sexual/romantic encounters. There is a reason why the most common definition of consent is the Planned Parenthood acronym FRIES (freely given, revocable, informed, enthusiastic, specific) (Planned Parenthood 2021). Consent is usually discussed in the same breath as sex. Consent seems to be a topic that everyone has heard of, but few have spent significant time exploring outside of a sexual context. When Elaine attended her son's college orientation in June 2022, the university's Title IX coordinator spoke for only five minutes, used the word "consent" only once, and only connected it to instances of avoiding forms of sexual advances and assault. No one else who spoke that day addressed consent. When consent and boundaries were introduced to a 300-level movement for the actor class at

Central Michigan University in Fall 2021, the response was overwhelming in that the students had never had a conversation about consent within a theatrical context before. They were shocked to be told that they are the only people who can make decisions about how their bodies are used and for what purposes. They had compartmentalized the consent information that some of them had been exposed to surrounding relationships and sex and did not consider that those same protocols apply to every moment of their everyday lives as well. If we were taught about consent from a very young age, the same way we're taught to learn that the cow says "moo" and the dog says "woof," we might live in a completely different culture. Why is learning to mimic the cow's voice more important than learning to use our own?

According to Cornell Law's Legal Information Institute, consent is "When a person voluntarily and willfully agrees to undertake an action that another person suggests" (LII/Legal Information Institute n.d.). Does this mean that consent isn't a consideration if the moment focuses on me undertaking an action I myself suggested? If I say I'll do something before someone else suggests it, do I have no recourse for withdrawing consent? According to the American Medical Association's Code of Medical Ethics, "The process of informed consent occurs when communication between a patient and physician results in the patient's authorization or agreement to undergo a specific medical intervention" (American Medical Association 2016). Does this mean that informed consent is not actively practiced unless it results in consent being granted? Or that "consent" refers specifically to an affirmative response? The homepage for CMU's Office of Civil Rights and Institutional Equity states "At CMU Consent means an affirmative, conscious decision by a participant to engage in sexual activity" (CMichSitefinity n.d.). The FDA even has their own definition of informed consent regarding participation in clinical trials (Office of the Commissioner 2020).

Merriam-Webster defines consent in two entries. The first entry: "to give assent or approval," the second entry: "compliance in or approval of what is done or proposed by another." (There is that external initiation of action again.) *Merriam-Webster* then lists "acquiescence" as a synonym that it defines as "passive acceptance and submission," which brings us to the problem of passivity having any place in active consent practices (Merriam-webster.com 2019). The Belmont Report, which addresses ethical issues to be considered when conducting research with human subjects, identifies the process of consent as having three components: "information, comprehension, and voluntariness" (The Belmont Report 1979: 10). A comprehensive disclosure of what's going to happen during the research in a manner (or manners) comprehensible to the potential participant, the potential participant's clear understanding of that information, and the participant's autonomous willingness to participate in what has been disclosed are all required.

These definitions, while delivering similar messages and having some minimally overlapping language, are distinct enough to not be interchangeable due to their specificity to the context of how consent lives within the institution that houses the definition. None of these individual definitions are appropriate for our needs in a performing arts context although they do each speak to aspects of the function of consent. Language makes the discussion of consent more challenging because it brings along with it suppositions, assumptions, individual frames of reference, and the like which can't be universally interpreted. There is a component of the personal interwoven with consent which can't be quantified in consistent language because it lives uniquely in each of us and in each of our experiences.

Recent, more mainstream discussions about consent practices in performance have been focused on the emerging fields of intimacy direction (live theatre) and intimacy coordination (film and television). This is where we began our discussion of consent in educational performance spaces. Our original research sought to expand that scope to introduce consent practices into the university dance studio, but it became clear over time that the work is applicable and, in fact, necessary across all performing arts disciplines. When discussing consent practices in performing arts classrooms and rehearsal spaces, we are not only talking about consent to touch, but, in the case of physical, emotional, and mental boundaries, consent to engage in a particular way with the material.

Consent is active, ongoing, and inherently communicative. It is the continuous navigation of a conversation about where individual boundaries lie and how they can be upheld, respected, and accommodated. According to *Ethics of Touch*,

> Boundaries separate people from their environment and other people. They are elusive, yet personally discernible, lines that distinguish you from everything and everyone around you. They define your personal space [...] Boundaries are not only physical, though. They also protect emotions and thoughts. Boundaries provide a sense of safety. They help you to sense how close or far away you want people, both physically and emotionally. Often you're unaware of your boundaries unless they're threatened or crossed.
>
> (Benjamin and Sohnen-Moe 2021a: 27)

While *Ethics of Touch* was originally written for somatic practitioners (chiropractors, massage therapists, physical therapists, etc.), many of its ideas translate readily to the performing arts.

> This concept may seem too obvious to mention, but many practitioners and organizations treat clients in depersonalizing ways to varying degrees. Healthcare

offices' procedures are often designed to make things easier for the organization or the practitioners, rather than to help put clients at ease.

(Benjamin and Sohnen-Moe 2021b: 91)

Many educators with more rigid or single-tracked teaching styles have established procedures that streamline or simplify their work but aren't necessarily the best methods for fostering productivity and growth in their students. If our goal is to assist each student in reaching their individual potential, it follows that we would need to employ an individualized approach: a foundation of standards and expectations, opportunities and goals for the students, and then a myriad of options for how to help them each reach their potential.

In our work as performing arts educators, we are obligated to care for the well-being of our students while they are in our charge. Yes, we need to encourage them to explore, to discover, to develop, and to grow, but we also need to do all of that ethically and responsibly. "Ethics are a set of principles and guidelines to help individuals make choices in order to avoid doing harm while working with others" (Bailey and Dickinson 2018: 225). We need to keep in mind that the end goal is not to get them to do what we're asking of them but to set them up for long-term success in a performing arts career. "Toughen up," "it's not that big a deal," "don't be so sensitive," "it's part of the job" are all dismissive, disengaged responses to student concerns. When students articulate that they are uncomfortable with some facet of their work, they need to be guided in exploring and assessing the discomfort, not told that the discomfort is somehow not real, not real enough, not valid, or not allowable. This requires us to have in place a regiment of routine which incorporates consent practices that genuinely hold space for our students to make choices about the way they work without repercussion or reprimand if they need to make a choice that we don't believe to be the best choice for them. We walk a blurry line of engaging students in a way that guides them forward in their development without finding ourselves behind them pushing or forcing that forward momentum. Later in the book, in the chapter on classroom facilitation, we discuss ways to guide students' exploration and assessment of their own boundaries in order to shepherd them forward in their growth as curious, mindful artists.

Fundamentally, our work can't be done ethically unless we respect each student and their autonomy. Always. No exceptions. This means that there will be times when students don't engage in the way *we'd* prefer. This means that we may disagree with how far students are willing to go in a particular activity/exercise/performance. This means that we may not see students reach the potential we believe to be waiting for them. And we must be okay with that. Education is not something you can force onto or into anyone. Our job is to offer with purpose and care and respect. We can't control whether the students choose to accept that offering, or how they choose to accept it, or how much or little of it they choose to accept. Our energies belong squarely focused on how to best facilitate the offering itself.

We also need to acknowledge that inextricably woven into consent-forward practices are robust practices targeting inclusivity and equity. In order to value and respect individual autonomy, we must acknowledge the experiences and frames of reference that each person brings to the shared space. "For individuality to flourish, teachers and trainers need to develop an understanding of how to embrace and play with difference in rehearsal and teaching settings and to move their focus away from a 'one approach fits all' mentality" (Hay and Landon-Smith 2018: 162). Additionally, the vastness that is our student body's experience cannot equitably be served by that mentality. As Chels Morgan states in their article "Visions for justice and critiquing consent: On taking performativity out of performance" in the *Journal of Consent Based Practices*,

> "safer" to one person is not and cannot be guaranteed as "safer" for another. In the same way, tools for consent that work for one person or one community cannot be guaranteed to yield the same results for those of us who live with compounded trauma and who are members of communities that thrive in their ambiguity.
> (Morgan 2022: 82)

Consent-forward work is predicated on acknowledging and honoring the uniqueness of each person and each person's experiences. This allows for those experiences to be part of the individual's autonomous decision-making process. As Zev Steinrock stated, "You can't have an inclusive space without it being consent-based. You also can't have a consent-based space without inclusive practices. They're intertwined" (Steinrock 2022).

Keep in mind that these practices aren't only in place for our students. They are in place to establish and safeguard our boundaries as educators as well. (Yes! We get to have our boundaries cared for too!) If you need to establish that you do not open, read, respond to e-mail on Saturdays, or between 9 p.m. and 7 a.m., put that in your syllabus. If you don't feel comfortable having closed-door meetings with students, post a notice right on your office door. If grade disputes must be discussed in person, share that information clearly. Respecting each human's autonomy means respecting ourselves, too.

Power Dynamics

There are any number of obstacles for our students to overcome as they begin their university education. In addition to being on their own for the first time in their lives, they may also carry personal experiences of trauma, neglect, or indifference as they walk in on day one. While we can't prepare for every possible type of student, we can have varied methodologies and training at the ready to work to accommodate diverse student needs. Most performing arts educators are not trained as mental health professionals and are not equipped to treat mental health challenges onsite, but we can work to mitigate the obstacle that we take part in creating: power dynamics. Susanne Shawyer and Kim Shively state, "Because power discrepancies can result in exploitative practices, it makes sense that theatre programs training students for the industry should prepare students to encounter hierarchies, and faculty should acknowledge how everyone in the room participates in structures of power" (Shawyer and Shively 2019: 90). Although this statement directly refers to theatre, the same holds true for all performing arts education.

According to French and Raven, there are six bases of power that could be at play in any given situation: legitimate, informational, expert, reward, referent, and coercive (French and Raven 1959: 150–67). As the authority figure in the classroom and/or rehearsal space, we automatically create legitimate power; there is a formal student–teacher relationship which places the teacher in the position of power as we create the content, run the room, and oversee the daily emotional climate of the space. This type of influence is based solely on our title or position, not necessarily on who we are as an individual. Our legitimate power as a professor teaching in our discipline doesn't exist for us when we're at home with a spouse, or at a parent–teacher conference for one of our children, or even in another classroom where the subject is something outside of our field of study. Legitimate power is based on the role we play in the room, not on who we are personally.

There is an informational base of power at play as teachers control the flow of information that reaches the students in order for them to achieve their learning objectives. We have what they need, and it is within our control to share generously or withhold greedily. It is within our control to share information with some students rather than with all students, and any number of variations on that theme. While the information we hold is not confidential (as it may be in an extreme case of informational power), it is usually solely ours until we make the decision to share it with the students. They are, after all, there to learn what we know.

We teach and train in higher education as specialists and experts in our fields. Incoming students assume that we know a whole lot more than they do. If they didn't, why would they invest the time and money in studying with us? That puts us in a position of power in any space that we share with our students. They are more likely to defer to our ideas, opinions, and suggestions simply because they believe us to be experts; we must know more and best. Not only do we assign grades (well, they earn grades, but they think we assign them), but in the performing arts, we are also their conductors, directors, choreographers, and project supervisors, and we have the ability to choose or not choose them for varying roles in productions and performances. They need letters of recommendation, references for scholarships, information from our network of professionals about internships, etc. Their work in the classroom is an ongoing audition for potential work outside of the classroom.

As the person running the room, most of us rely, to some degree, on referent power. We work to forge connection and trust in order to foster the student's ability to settle into the space and engage more deeply in their own learning. When they can see their teacher, their mentor, their director as an approachable supporter, someone who can help, someone who is genuinely invested in their progress, they are more likely to genuinely invest in their own progress as well.

In his book *Nonviolent Communication*, Marshall B. Rosenberg has several pages dedicated to the feelings that come up for us when our needs are being met vs. when they are not. When they're not being met, for example we may feel "ashamed [...] confused [...] discouraged [...] embarrassed [...] hostile [...] lonely [...] unsteady [...] withdrawn." When they are being met, we may feel "adventurous ... curious ... encouraged [...] free [...] hopeful [...] inspired [...] joyful [...] proud [...] secure [...] wide-awake" (Rosenberg 2015: 44–46). When we teach in a manner that fosters the feelings in the second list, we can help to create a space where the students can do their best work; we open them up to the ability to tap into their own power. Nicole Perry reminds us that "[w]e don't empower students. Students already have power. We simply create opportunities for them to step into it, to practice it. Or not" (Perry 2022). We can choose to cultivate an environment where the student can flex their autonomy and state their needs, concerns, boundaries, and ideas with the confidence of knowing that there will be support, respect, and even admiration for that flex.

Now, it would be ideal to say that no arts educator uses coercive power in the classroom, but given our own experiences and those shared with us by colleagues and students around the country, we know that is simply not true. We know that some educators have used their power to get what they want rather than to give the students the education they need. We also know that some of us have unknowingly overstepped our boundaries with students as a result of one or more of these power bases being present. Mistakes have been made. Mistakes will continue to be made. As long as we're not avoiding apologies and repeating those same mistakes rather than learning from them, we can continue to walk along the road to progress. (We talk more about owning our mistakes and modeling apologies in the activities section of this book.)

In addition to power dynamics, there is also the principle of the power paradox delineated by Dacher Keltner. In his book, *The Power Paradox, How We Gain and Lose Influence*, Keltner states that

> the seductions of power induce us to lose the very skills that enabled us to gain power in the first place [...] By succumbing to the power paradox, we undermine

our own power and cause others, on whom our power so critically depends, to feel threatened and devalued.

(Keltner 2016a: 9)

He discusses the nature of power and how we receive it from others based on a sustained focus on others, and how we lose it when our focus turns inward to the self. Later in his book, the cost of powerlessness is discussed as both physical and mental.

> Powerlessness is the most robust trigger of stress and cortisol release [...] Chronic threat and stress orient the individual toward defense, undermining most other ways of engaging in the world and causing problems with sleep, sex, creative thought, and trusting interactions with others. Chronic threat and stress damage regions of the brain that are involved in planning and the pursuit of goals.
>
> (Keltner 2016b: 141)

This is important to keep in mind as educators: when we maintain a clear focus on student-centered learning and working in the best interest of our students, we do our best in creating a space where they feel valued. That self-value builds confidence and emboldens students to step into their own power in order to do their best work risking, failing, trying, and growing.

Co-existing with the teacher–student power dynamic present in the space, there are any number of additional power dynamic considerations that create structures and influence the way students engage and make decisions. The student–student dynamic can be influenced by the combinations of upper- and under-class levels (perceived expertise), the overall makeup of the people in the space in terms of the intersectionalities of student identities, competition for similar roles or opportunities, the desire to work with (or not work with) certain classmates, etc. Working to mitigate the teacher–student power dynamics can also provide some amelioration to those that already exist between and amongst our students.

So, take a moment if you will and consider the following: How did power play a role in your arts education? Can you remember a time when you felt like you had no power to make decisions freely? How did that experience live within you? And now, as you recall it, how does it show up? What could your mentor(s) have done to better serve you in those moments of powerlessness? Maintain that student lens as you shift your focus to today and consider the sort of power you have and feel in the space you're privileged to run. Is it serving your students? How can you work to make the important adjustment from having power over your students to developing power with your students? What will it take to begin the move away from control and toward collaboration?

Verbal and Non-verbal Consent

Further complicating our work is the issue of how consent can be communicated. The long-standing "No Means No" slogan doesn't really speak to the complexities of how we communicate in a moment when we are giving, withholding, or withdrawing consent. While verbal cues of "yes" or "no" are perhaps the clearest methods, we habitually speak in all sorts of combinations of slang, gesture, and expression that give our everyday speech nuance. How often do we actually say "yes" when someone asks if we want to do something? More often, we respond with a version of the yes, "yeah, sure," "okay," "alright." Alternatively (or additionally), we may shrug our shoulders, move our head, slowly blink our eyes and smile a bit, or provide any number of nonverbal signals that might tell someone we're giving consent. As with vernacular, we each bring our own interpretive frames of reference to deciphering nonverbal cues, and some of us have lots of trouble reading nonverbal cues at all. The tone of my voice when I say "okay" may clearly indicate that I don't actually want to say yes, that I feel scared, hesitant, or pressured to do so. A different tone may clearly convey enthusiasm. "Where there is confusion, people are more likely to interpret what they're seeing as being in line with what they want" (Surmick et al. 2019: 54). We need to be mindful of receiving verbal cues, nonverbal cues, and combinations of both in order to most effectively interpret what is being communicated. This requires that we are alert and attentive to our students as we communicate, and that we objectively assess the responses we receive rather than preemptively forcing them to conform with our preferred responses.

This brings us to the single greatest consent issue that we face as educators: our students are never in a position to truly give consent. We can acknowledge and address power dynamics. We can tell our students that we value their autonomy and that they should too. We can foster an environment that encourages students to speak their truths, but we can never actually remove the power dynamics and the impact they have on the people in the space. This means that the student–teacher hierarchy will always remain intact and that the student will never be completely free from the effects of those power bases described by French and Raven. Something that we need to share with students when discussing consent is the limitation of our best efforts. Our best efforts are just that: the best we can do in that particular moment and situation. The keys to creating an environment in which students can step into their power and autonomy are communication and transparency. Letting students know that we will fall short does not weaken our position and in fact could help to create a stronger educational community.

Resistance to Incorporating Consent Practices

There are certainly educators and professionals in the performing arts who are uninterested in implementing these practices. While there are any number of reasons this may be the case, there appear to be two primary reasons. First, these folks seem to feel that we're out to strip their existing practices and pedagogy away and build anew from the ground up. That's not at all the case. No one is out to erase another professional's experience and wisdom. We just want to move forward in a more effective way that provides robust support for our students' physical and mental well-being. In order to make change, we must objectively reflect on our current practices and that may be a scary process. As we were reminded by Betty Martin in both her book, *The Art of Receiving and Giving: The Wheel of Consent*, and the interview (Martin 2023) we conducted with her, there are risks to the work of investigating and reflecting on consent forward practices. "There is always a risk in increasing your awareness. You risk seeing things you might rather not notice" (Martin 2021: 5). While this is absolutely true, the potentially risky reflection allows us to add important new tools to our long-standing toolkits which may better serve our students.

Second, some practitioners see it as an easy out for the students. Common responses of resistance are "this just gives students a way to not have to participate," "what happens when no one feels like engaging in the work," or "they're not going to have that choice once they're working professionally." In our experience, and the experiences of those interviewed, few if any students see consent-based work as an "out." In fact, the opposite has proven to be true. Students are hungry for this and are engaging more deeply in their explorations because the spaces in which they learn and work are putting their well-being at the top of the priority list. A single student who may abuse this process as a way to back out of work they just don't want to do is probably a student who would've found another way to back out of participating anyway. A student consistently pulling away from engaging in work simply because they have the option to do so is a student who likely isn't in possession of the rigorous self-discipline and desire for personal growth required to be successful. We can't say no to facilitating consent-forward practices because a few students may abuse it. The practices will still be of enormous benefit to most.

Finally, if respecting autonomy and engaging in active consent practices is not part of the professional experience, isn't it our ethical duty as educators to assist in creating that change? If we instill those fundamental expectations in our students, they will carry them into the professional world year after year, graduating class after graduating class, until performing arts professions are full of people with those same expectations and standards. Our work with students in higher education can have an enormous impact on how our professional industries operate. The graduates of our programs will have toolkits full of not just what we taught them, but how we taught it. We are training our future colleagues, and that is how we make the industry better for everyone.

A Connection to Power Dynamics That We Can't Ignore

We would be remiss if we didn't address the additional complication of the experiences of the past few years related to the COVID-19 pandemic. The direct and indirect exposure to the virus and its repercussions has left indelible marks on our bodies and minds. As our students have navigated their way through the pandemic, they've been masked and distanced, masked without distance, unmasked and distanced, and other combinations of these options. As their teachers, we've made these transitions with them but without the informational power that we usually possess. Just like them, we've had little to no information about what the days ahead would hold and how we'd deal with those ever-changing circumstances. This parallel experience also contributed to shifting power dynamics as we attempted to do the thing we've always done without really fully knowing how we were going to do it. We certainly felt lost. We suddenly felt like we no longer knew how to teach. Our skill sets felt weakened stripped, exhausted, and forcefully challenged. Simultaneously, we were also losing our grip on our interpersonal skill set which forced us to physically engage (or not engage) in completely new ways both in our long-term, well-established relationships and in the brand-new relationships we were attempting to forge with new students. We were hand-sanitizing constantly, shutting our homes to visitors, scrubbing our groceries, and becoming suspicious of the proximity of others. Our average, every day stress was elevated to unsustainable levels and we were still trying to control that narrative and protect our students from it. What we didn't realize right away was that it wasn't something that needed to be kept from students. Our struggles and our uncertainties became a sort of salve for the students' struggles; once they understood that we were in a shared experience some of the uncertainty lost its scariness, its tension, and its power over all of us. *Lesson learned: Our vulnerabilities are not inherently negative and our ability to share them can be a tool for facilitating growth and building community.*

Despite that positive outcome, we are all moving forward with the weight of the past few years dragging behind us. Even as we excitedly look to a future that allows us to regain some type of normalcy (whatever that is) we are not free from the pandemic. Some of us are dealing with serious long-term complications from having had COVID, some are grieving the loss of loved ones (either from COVID or during a time when we were unable to gather and say goodbye in the way we'd have wanted), and others are suffering the continued frustrations of managing interpersonal relationships with people who deny, refuse, and otherwise painfully strain the relationship. Some recent studies have even shown that the COVID pandemic has caused PTSD-like symptoms in people who never had COVID. A study by Bridgland et al. out of Flinders University in Australia found that participants had "PTSD-like symptoms for events that had not yet happened, challenging the nature of traumatic stress as a problem pertaining only to the past" (Bridgland et al. 2021: n.pag.). Participants showed classic markers of stress related to the *anticipation of* potential COVID-related traumatic experiences looming in their future. So we're not only processing the difficulties we've already experienced as a result of the global pandemic, many of us are also grappling with what may still happen. Any way you look at it, whether the student is consciously aware that all of this is present or not, that's a whole lot of additional pressure to manage every Monday, Wednesday, and Friday at 9 a.m.

REFERENCES

American Medical Association (2016), "Informed consent," https://www.ama-assn.org/delivering-care/ethics/informed-consent. Accessed 20 June 2022.

Baczynski, M. and Scott, E. (2022), *Creating Consent Culture*, London and Philadelphia, PA: Jessica Kingsley Publishers, p. 31.

Bailey, S. and Dickinson, P. (2018), "Generating ethics and social justice in applied theatre curricula," in A. Fliotsos and G. S. Medford (eds), *New Directions in Teaching Theatre Arts*, Cham: Palgrave Macmillan, pp. 225–48.

Benjamin, B. E. and Sohnen-Moe, C. (2021a), *The Ethics of Touch: The Hands-on Practitioner's Guide to Creating a Professional, Safe, and Enduring Practice*, Tucson, AZ: Sma, Sohnen Moe Associates, Inc., p. 27.

Benjamin, B. E. and Sohnen-Moe, C. (2021b), *The Ethics of Touch: The Hands-on Practitioner's Guide to Creating a Professional, Safe, and Enduring Practice*, Tucson, AZ: Sma, Sohnen Moe Associates, Inc., p. 91.

Bridgland, V. M. E., Moeck, E. K., Green, D. M., Swain, T. L., Nayda, D. M., Matson, L. A., Hutchison, N. P. and Takarangi, M. K. T. (2021), "Why the COVID-19 pandemic is a traumatic stressor," *PLOS ONE*, 16:1, p. e0240146.

CMichSitefinity (n.d.), "Glossary of sexual and gender-based misconduct terms," https://www.cmich.edu/offices-departments/OCRIE/title-ix-sexual-gender-based-misconduct/glossary-sexual-gender-based-misconduct-terms. Accessed 30 June 2022.

Commissioner, O. of the (2020), "Informed consent," U.S. Food and Drug Administration, https://www.fda.gov/regulatory-information/search-fda-guidance-documents/informed-consent#summayrproc. Accessed 20 June 2022.

"consent" (2019), Merriam-Webster, https://www.merriam-webster.com/dictionary/consent. Accessed 5 June 2022.

French, J. R. P., Jr. and Raven, B. (1959), "The bases of social power," in D. Cartwright (ed.), *Studies in Social Power*, Ann Arbor, MI: University of Michigan, pp. 150–67.

Hay, C. and Landon-Smith, K. (2018), "The intercultural actor: Embracing difference in theatre arts teaching," in A. Fliotsos and G. S. Medford (eds), *New Directions in Teaching Theatre Arts*, Cham: Palgrave Macmillan, pp. 157–73.

Keltner, D. (2016a), *The Power Paradox: How We Gain and Lose Influence*, New York, NY: Penguin Books, p. 9.

Keltner, D. (2016b), *The Power Paradox: How We Gain and Lose Influence*, New York, NY: Penguin Books, p. 141.

LII / Legal Information Institute (n.d.), "Consent," https://www.law.cornell.edu/wex/consent. Accessed 20 June 2022.

Martin, B. (2021), *The Art of Receiving and Giving: The Wheel of Consent*, Eugene, OR: Luminare Press, p. 5.

Martin, B. (2023), interviewed by E. Daugherty and H. Trommer-Beardslee, Online 3 July 2023.

Morgan, C. (2022), "Visions for justice and critiquing consent: On taking performativity out of performance," *The Journal of Consent Based Practices*, 1:2, pp. 80–110, https://journals.calstate.edu/jcbp/article/view/2870/2989. Accessed 28 July 2023.

Perry, N. (2022), interviewed by E. Daugherty and H. Trommer-Beardslee, Online 4 May 2022.

Planned Parenthood (2021), "What is sexual consent? / Facts about rape & sexual assault," https://www.plannedparenthood.org/learn/relationships/sexual-consent. Accessed 30 June 2022.

Rosenberg, M. (2015), *Nonviolent Communication: A Language of Life*, Encinitas, CA: PuddleDancer Press, pp. 44–46.

Shawyer, S. and Shively, K. (2019), "Education in theatrical intimacy as ethical practice for University Theatre," *Journal of Dramatic Theory and Criticism*, 34:1, pp. 87–104.

Steinrock, Z. (2022), interviewed by E. Daugherty and H. Trommer-Beardslee, Online 26 May 2022.

Surmick, S. Drake, R., Monroe, L., O'Hanlon, K. and Hirsch, L. (2019), *The Consent Primer: Foundations for Everyday Life*, Seattle, WA: The Consent Academy, A Part of the Pan Eros Foundation, p. 54.

The Belmont Report (1979), *Ethical Principles and Guidelines for the Protection of Human Subjects in Research*, p. 10, https://babel.hathitrust.org/cgi/pt?id=mdp.39015004406214& view=1up&seq=1. Accessed 14 July 2023.

2

Programmatic Policies

For faculty and administrators, especially those in creative and performance-driven spaces, approaching the profession from the position of empathetic heart and mind work will positively contribute to equity-driven engagement and improved learning dynamics [...] Ultimately, this approach enhances student performance outcomes, because the practice allows students to feel and know they are safe while learning, exploring, and creating in a non-threatening or harmful environment.

Jasmine D. Parker (2022: 49)

In the summer of 2022, we conducted an IRB-approved anonymous online survey on touch practices in performing arts classrooms that was distributed to our professional contacts and national performing arts organizations who then distributed the survey link further. The 60 respondents represented the following disciplines:

Music: 10.91%
Theatre: 20%
Dance: 63.64%
Other: 5.45%

Within these disciplines, the respondents indicated that they work for the following categories of establishments:

Private lessons/self-employed: 16.47%
Community organization: 10.59%
Private/Independent business: 22.35%
K-12 education: 15.29%
Higher education: 35.29%
Other: 0%

When asked if they use touch (physical contact between teacher and student) as an instructional tool or as a method of correction in their courses, 90.2% of the survey respondents answered yes and 9.8% responded no. When asked if any of the course content included touch (physical contact between students), 72.55% of the respondents answered yes and 27.45% of the respondents answered no. Then, when asked if they have established consent practices (consent to be touched) in their courses, 64.71% of the respondents answered yes and 35.29% answered no. When asked to expand on the nature of the practices, the respondents described syllabus language, verbal consent, class discussions, check-ins, google forms, and parent meetings. While these percentages reflect a very small sampling of performing arts educators, the numbers do reflect a need for consent-based practices. While 90.2% of respondents use touch, only 64.71% have consent practices associated with the use of touch and the robustness of those practices is not clear.

Across the board, practices can streamline the way we approach and interact with students in every space related to coursework, practicums, and productions. While university-wide codes of conduct may address issues of consent, they are usually directly connected to sexual assault and harassment. We know from our own experiences and those of interviewed colleagues that students don't necessarily extrapolate that information and apply it to other facets of their lives. An official statement of commitment to consent-based practices for a whole program and each faculty and staff member who works within that program can serve as a foundation for expectations across the disciplines. Whether you are a dance department, a music department, or a school of performing arts that houses music, dance, and theatre, establishing standards for behavior that are published and accessible creates transparency, and can soften the harsh edges of power structures by letting students see that there are expectations for how their teachers and mentors will behave.

A statement of the department's commitment can live right on the program's website and within foundational marketing literature. This is the most transparent approach. Whenever anyone researches your program, the fact that the entire program is committed to this consent-forward behavior is made known. This can be reassuring for prospective students and their families, potential faculty or staff applicants, and guest artists considering your program for a fixed-term post or residency. This commitment speaks to the overall approach to human interaction. As Donna Freitas stated in *Consent on campus: a manifesto*, "prioritizing consent is also prioritizing a set of ethics [...] it is a way of *being toward others*. By creating a set of ethical expectations and values that reflect this, we can create a culture of consent" (Freitas 2018: 135). This can be reinforced by including the statement in syllabi for the program's courses. When students see this, they understand that not only are these the standards for the program as a whole, but you personally will be upholding them in the learning spaces that you have the privilege of running. Again, this offers reassurance to students right from the moment the course begins that you have established standards for how everyone will be treating each other—you included. We will unpack this in more detail when we discuss individual classroom practices.

A programmatic policy will be most helpful and most effective if it is collaboratively created by the group of people who will be expected to uphold it. "While it starts at the top, leadership is a quality that extends through every level of an organization. The responsibility to change a culture must be shared throughout the whole" (Bellinger et al. 2022). Because our world, our programs, and our students' needs are ever-changing, the policy can be put on the department's agenda once a year to open up conversation about what may need to be revised or updated in order to best serve the needs of the program. Investing in the creation of the expectations will likely increase buy-in which is essential since the policy is not something that can be implemented without the full commitment of the individual members of the program. A major problem with these public statements can arise if they are solely performative. That is, the statement is crafted and made available for the sake of saying that a statement has been crafted and made available, but no real action is taken to hold the members of the program accountable for living up to the established expectations. There needs to be action that backs up the statement to make it clear that this is a way of behaving, not simply an abstract idea. This takes the form of our daily interactions with students in classrooms, rehearsal spaces, advising sessions, and even casual or impromptu "hallway meetings" that happen without planning. These interactions need to be underpinned and guided by the program policy and backed up with a clear chain of reporting for when we fall short of those expectations. There is a long history of businesses using hierarchical flow charts in order to create a clear system of communication for problem-solving purposes. The founders of Theatrical Intimacy Education, Laura Rikard and Chelsea Pace, applied this systematic structure to the performing arts and included process-based information in *Staging Sex; Best Practices, Tools, and Techniques for Theatrical Intimacy*. "The Chain of Communication is a document that outlines the best practices for communicating concerns in a process" (Pace and Rikard 2020: 101). In our June 2023 interview, Rikard explained that at TIE, they use the word "communication" as opposed to "reporting" because "reporting makes it sound like a chain of policing and that is not what it is; it is not a snitch chain. It is a method of communicating when there are concerns. It is not about going over someone's head" (Rikard et al. 2023).

This chain can vary from space to space and situation to situation. In its most basic form, the chain provides information about who an individual can go to in the event that boundaries are breached, or expectations are not upheld. For a university classroom, this structure may include professors, department chairs, college deans, and leaders in Diversity, Equity, and Inclusion (DEI), and Title IX. Within a production, the structure may include stage managers, directors, choreographers, intimacy directors, and music directors. Chains can be created as flow charts that visually show steps from incident to communication to resolution or can be written out in paragraph form to explain the available options.

A chain of communication tells students that while you may be the authority figure in the room, you are not the only authority figure they can engage. If we do something in class that breaches the boundaries of a student, our hope is that we've created a culture where they feel they can speak directly to us in the moment that it happens. That is not always the case for any number of reasons. This chain lets them know that if they are not comfortable speaking directly to us, they can speak to another professor in the program, or the chair of the department, or whoever else it may be appropriate to include in that chain. It gives the student options, and lets them know that our work is overseen by others who hold us to the established standards; that outside the classroom or rehearsal space we are in spaces where we do not hold the legitimate power. When students are made aware of the vulnerabilities of our power, it can provide an additional safeguard that may allow them to engage more productively in the work.

We asked Mary Martinez, the Title IX coordinator at Central Michigan University, to provide some guidance in terms of language to use and language to avoid when crafting a policy. She suggested the following (Martinez 2022):

- make sure it references the university-wide policy (to bolster your policy with support)
- avoid victimizing language
- use "complainant" rather than "victim" for the person bringing the complaint forward
- use "respondent" rather than "accused" for the person responding to the complaint
- avoid "you" language as in "you must report …" which can sound accusatory and create additional, undue pressure
- use "options are …" and/or list whatever resources are available
- be mindful of the tone of the writing-use inclusive language and inclusive pronouns (rather than having policy assume victim/female, accused/male)
- include info about mandatory reporting.

Samples of Programmatic Policies

We have excerpted some pieces of policy below for two reasons. First, to show that there is already department- and program-wide policy in place in various institutions that articulate commitment to consent practices and the equity and inclusion that are foundational to its success. The work is happening. You are not alone in wanting to make this happen for your program and these resources may help bolster your pursuit of investment in this work from colleagues who may be hesitant. Second, these can serve as jumping-off points and conversation starters as you work to craft the policy that will best serve the needs of your program.

The inclusion of materials here should not be assumed to mean that the writing/intention/language contained within them is "right." There is no one right way to do this, so the examples are varied (some extensive, some just a bullet point that really resonated with us) with the hope that they can provide a spark of inspiration regardless of your needs. Some policies included below are readily available on institution websites, others are internal documents that have been shared with permission.

The Boston Conservatory at Berklee's Theater Division shared their program policies with us and we've excerpted them below. "Guidelines" include information on how mistakes are handled and the chain of reporting in cases of violations. "Community Practices" includes language that specifically outlines how touch will be handled in both classroom and performance spaces.

(Excerpt from "Guidelines")

- Mistakes and failure are part of the process. Allow others to realize and take responsibility for them. Give feedback with learning as a goal rather than chastising or calling out. Take feedback from another person regarding language, process, or work as intended to help rather than criticize.
- Classroom accommodations will be provided in partnership with Accessibility Services.
- If there is a violation of community standards, it should be brought to a faculty member, program leadership, or division administration, and/or the proper institutional office.

(Excerpt from "Community Practices")

1. There will be performed no violence, intimate contact, sexual violence, or simulated sex without specific choreography and consent-based rehearsal.
2. There will be no nudity in work in the classroom, in curricular projects, or in student-directed work. Nudity in faculty-directed projects will be handled with best practices and consent, and students will be notified on the audition forms of the desire of inclusion of nudity.
3. Consent will be sought before physical contact and consent can be withdrawn at any point in the process by anyone.

Kimberley Cooper, artistic director of Decidedly Jazz Danceworks in Calgary, shared their company disclosures which include "Respectful Workplace" and "Dancer Policies." The first document is shared with anyone who joins the organization for the first time. The second is part of a policy handbook given to each member of the dance company on an annual basis.

(Excerpt from "Respectful Workplace")

What are my responsibilities?
All DJD employees, dancers, contractors, volunteers, and students are responsible for keeping our environment free of discrimination and harassment. We are responsible for maintaining a respectful workplace by complying with the policy and ensuring our behavior meets the standards set out in this policy. We are also responsible for taking appropriate action (as outlined below) if we witness harassing incidents. When management or directors become aware that discrimination or harassment may have occurred, they are obligated by law to take prompt and appropriate action, whether or not the individual targeted wants DJD to do so. Under no circumstances should a complaint be dismissed or downplayed.

What should I do if I feel I'm being harassed?
Address the Issue Directly: Employees, dancers, contractors, volunteers, and students are encouraged to attempt to resolve their concerns through direct communication with the person(s) engaging in the unwelcome conduct. Where employees, dancers, contractors, volunteers, or students feel confident or comfortable in doing so, communicate disapproval in clear terms to the person(s) whose conduct or comments are offensive. Keep a written record of the date, time, details of the conduct, and witnesses, if any. Usually, this approach resolves the conflict. Where the individual is uncomfortable directly approaching the person(s) engaging in improper or offensive behaviour, or where the individual's direct approach has not resolved their concerns, a facilitated discussion is recommended.

Facilitated Support and Intervention
Employees, dancers, contractors, volunteers, or students who are not confident or comfortable with the approach to address the issue directly as described above and who believe they are victims of discrimination or harassment or become aware of situations where such conduct may be occurring, are encouraged to report these matters to the Executive Director, the Artistic Director or Board Chair.

This information is reiterated in the "Safety" section of their "Dancer Policies" document.

(Excerpt from "Dancer Policies")

The Dancers' safety and security are of utmost importance. Please read the Respectful Workplace Policy. In dance, lines of touching and safety regarding movement can be ambiguous. Should the Dancer feel uncomfortable speaking up in the moment, please speak to the Artistic Director or Rehearsal Director as soon as possible.

Mental health is as important as physical health. There are counseling services in our building.

(Calgary Counseling Centre 2022)

The online student handbook for the American Conservatory Theater in San Francisco includes the following bullet point on the work of actor training. It is a short and sweet reminder that the student is autonomous and that the distinction between discomfort and fear should be critically assessed.

Actor training will stretch your boundaries. However, you are the author of your own training: you may say 'stop' whenever you feel you cannot pursue a particular line further. At the same time, challenging yourself and saying 'yes' to your creative work whenever possible leads to growth. Saying 'no' should not be used as an "excuse."

On the "Student Resources" page of Utah Valley University's Department of Theatrical Arts for Stage & Screen, there is a link to the program's "Touch, Boundaries, and Consent" policy. This resource lays out guidelines for student–student interactions, for student–teacher interactions, and for the process of selecting material. Just beneath that link is "Communicating Concerns" which lays out the types of concerns that might warrant reporting as well as multiple pathways for facilitating that reporting. These pathways give students several options for how to move toward resolution with a note at the top of the page that states "you may enter this response network at any point that is comfortable for you, or at more than one point" (n.d.).

The following excerpt is from Yale School of Drama (YSD) Protocol for Rehearsing and Performing Material with Sexual Content, Consensual Sexual Touching, and Depicting Sexual Assault. This speaks directly to class work with heightened material and articulates the support of student autonomy as they move through the work. It clearly states the teacher's responsibility to honor the needs of the student and includes chain of reporting information should additional support be needed.

Responsibilities of Teachers

It is the responsibility of the teacher to alert students when they are assigned scene work that may involve consensual sexual touching, including kissing. Such notice may be given in writing, via e-mail, or during an in-person meeting with the stage manager and any involved scene partners. Best practices at YSD include contextualizing explorations of sexuality in the classroom. Students will acknowledge they understand that they are consenting to explore sexuality and/or consensual sexual touching.

Teachers will honor a student's right to pause during a scene, if the student feels unsafe. Teachers who have questions with respect to implementation of these protocols should contact the Chair of their department or Associate Dean/YSD Title IX Coordinator Chantal Rodriguez.

Arizona State University School of Music, Dance, and Theatre has a bullet point in their online DEI statement that specifically addresses their commitment to how they handle intimacy which centers consent practices in its work.

Provide training opportunities for students, faculty and staff in Intimacy staging, and engage Intimacy coordinators for productions where appropriate.

University of Maryland, Baltimore County has a program policy on their website that was developed by Chelsea Pace and the UMBC Theatre faculty and staff. Listed as a resource under the "Current Students" tab is the "Theatrical Intimacy and Instructional Touch Policy." The page outlines best practices and includes the following syllabus language:

The Theatre Department at UMBC is dedicated to integrating consent-based practices into all classroom and production environments. In all Theatre Department related activities, all participants are expected to abide by the Instructional Touch and Theatrical Intimacy Best Practices. All participants in UMBC Theatre activities are expected to communicate their boundaries, ask before they touch, and maintain a professional working environment. The full policy detailing the Best Practices is available on the department website.

The Department of Theatre and Dance at Central Michigan University collaboratively created a program policy in 2022. This is the language that is included on all course syllabi and may be accessed on our department webpage.

Arts environments require risk, courage, vulnerability, and investment of our physical, emotional, and intellectual selves.

(Not In Our House December 2017)

CMU's Department of Theatre and Dance pledges to nurture safety, respect, and accountability through the support of the agency of our students. Directors/choreographers, instructors, managers of employment, students, and others will endeavor to establish and respect physical, emotional, and professional boundaries while balancing the artistic and educational vision and needs of the production, class, and/or employment position. In our efforts to foster safe and caring environments, to increase transparency, and to encourage personal and community accountability, a clear process for concern resolution will be made available in all our spaces.

REFERENCES

American Conservatory Theater Student Handbook (n.d.), p. 9, https://www.act-sf.org/training/mfa/. Accessed 15 July 2022.

Arizona State University (n.d.), "Music theatre and opera diversity, equity and inclusion initiatives," Herberger Institute for Design and the Arts, School of Music, Dance and Theatre, https://musicdancetheatre.asu.edu/music-theatre-and-opera/diversity-equity-inclusion. Accessed 16 August 2022.

Bellinger, B. and Projection, Lights, and Staging News (2022), "Production on deck: Eliminating excuses," 4 February, https://plsn.com/articles/stage-directions-articles/production-on-deck-eliminating-excuses-2. Accessed 7 July 2023.

CMU, Central Michigan University (n.d.), College of the Arts and Media, Department of Theatre and Dance Consent Statement, https://www.cmich.edu/academics/colleges/college-arts-media/departments-schools/theatre-dance/about-the-department-of-theatre-and-dance. Accessed 19 August 2023.

Collins Bandes, P. (2022), unarchived source received.

Communicating Concerns Purpose (n.d.), *Student Handbook*, Utah Valley University, Department of Theatrical Arts for Stage and Screen, https://www.uvu.edu/theatre/docs/concern-communication-pathway.pdf. Accessed 6 August 2022.

Cooper, K. (2022), unarchived source received.

Freitas, D. (2018), *Consent on Campus: A Manifesto*, New York, NY: Oxford University Press, p. 135.

Martinez, M. (2022), interviewed by E. Daugherty and H. Trommer-Beardslee, Online 27 June 2022.

Not In Our House (2017), "#NotInOurHouse: A Chicago theatre community," https://www.notinourhouse.org/. Accessed 15 May 2022.

Pace, C. and Rikard, L. (2020), *Staging Sex: Best Practices, Tools, and Techniques for Theatrical Intimacy*, New York, NY: Routledge, p. 101.

Parker, J. (2022), "Transforming community and ourselves through heart and mind work: A pathway for embracing diversity, inclusion, equity, belonging, and justice," in M. Stepniak (ed.), *A More Promising Musical Future: Leading Transformational Change in Music Higher Education*, Abingdon: Taylor and Francis Group, pp. 37–61.

Rikard, L. (2023), interviewed by E. Daugherty and H. Trommer-Beardslee, Online 9 June 2023.

University of Maryland Baltimore County (n.d.), "Theatrical intimacy and instructional touch policy," Department of Theatre, https://theatre.umbc.edu/current-students/theatrical-intimacy-and-instructional-touch-policy/. Ratified 26 August 2019. Accessed 6 June 2023.

Yale College (n.d.), "Guidelines for rehearsing material with sexual content," Yale Undergraduate Production, https://up.yalecollege.yale.edu/policies/guidelines-rehearsing-material-sexual-content. Accessed 15 July 2022.

3

Classroom Facilitation

So, what sorts of practices do we need to implement in order to actionably support the policies outlined in Chapter Two? How can we integrate consent-forward work into our existing pedagogy? And/or can we objectively assess our existing pedagogy and insert this work into spaces vacated by practices that have overstayed their welcome and are no longer aligned with our values as educators? We must begin where all new skills begin: in discomfort. As the saying goes, the expert in anything was once a beginner. If we expect our students to step into newness, so must we if we truly want to change their experience for the better.

Assessment of existing pedagogy is the first step. As we stated previously, no one is asking that teachers throw away everything they've used in the past and start all over from scratch. No one needs to reinvent the wheel. We *do* need to see if these particular wheels are still capable of getting us where we want to go in the manner in which we now wish to travel.

Syllabi and Community Agreements

The course syllabus is a first point of contact for your students. If it is available and they are reading it before the first day of class, it is their first impression of you and your expectations. Historically, the syllabus has set the bar for rigor and established the power of the teacher over the student by outlining expected learning outcomes, assignments and deadlines, grading policies, and penalties for not meeting expectations. Since 2004, however, when Ken Bain introduced the "promising syllabus" in his book, *What the Best College Teachers Do*, many have been objectively reexamining their syllabi to see them from the students' perspective understanding that students will be more deeply invested in their education when they have some say in how it will unfold. Teachers are working to revamp the once strict and rigid course syllabus in order to create documents that focus on offering students pathways to learning rather than demanding that students learn in a particular prescribed way (Bain 2004).

Instructors, either as part of the syllabus or as a supplemental document, can also work with students to create class contracts or community agreements that evolve out of group discussion. These agreements lay out the expectations for each member of the group and articulate how the group will work both as individuals and as a collective to uphold those expectations and hold each other accountable. This is a wonderful way to develop understanding within the group and to immediately begin facilitating conversations not just about what the class will do but how the class will go about doing it. Artists do their best, most creative work when they are at ease in an environment that they perceive to be supportive and collaborative. With consistent consent-based practices integrated into the process, our student artists become part of the creation of a culture that allows them to do their best work. They are able to engage in the development of artistic work, yes, but also in the work of creating the agreed-upon container in which that artistic work is developed.

L.A.-based intimacy director, sex educator, theatre director, and community facilitator Carly DW Bones spoke of community agreements as "one of my favorite tools for harm reduction and prevention" (Bones 2022). By creating a list of action items/philosophical understandings together as a class or production group, the list acts as a commitment from everyone involved and can be relied upon throughout the entirety of the group's time together. Everyone has agency to uphold and care for the agreement created by the entire community. Community agreements are a living document. Nothing is set in stone, and agreements can change or be added to as needs come up throughout the process. These agreements are also a great way to build shared language to call people in with grace and compassion if they act outside of the agreements at any point in the process.

How to Create Community Agreements

You can start the process by asking the following questions:

How are we going to agree to show up and care for each other while making art/learning together?

What do we need to do (or how are we going to behave) in order to be successful as a group?

What does this group need to agree on in order to feel like they can show up to class/rehearsal and be in a brave space?

If these questions do not get the participants started on creating agreements, consider asking them to think about a time in which they had a learning experience that was very successful. What happened within the group that made the experience successful? How can that need/experience be translated to a community agreement? The opposite of this is asking students to think of a learning experience in which their needs were not met. This negative experience can be used to analyze what would have been helpful and can be translated to the community agreement to set the group up for success. The process for creating community agreements is typically as important as the product, the agreement, in terms of uniting a group of people to work toward a common goal, in this case productive learning. Taking the time early on to create a mindful culture in your classroom/rehearsal room is a powerful investment that will improve both the process and product.

Recently, Elaine used a community agreement in a special topics course. The idea was introduced on day one and students were asked to give some thought to what they would like to include so that there could be discussion to create a first draft in the following class session. The main question posed to them was, "How can we best show up with and for each other and ourselves?" At the beginning of the second class, the group brainstormed together to phrase their ideas in ways that were clear and understandable to the whole group and were given the option to submit ideas via e-mail if they did not want to speak up at the moment in class. Once the e-mailed ideas were added, the final agreement was shared with the group in the following class and it was agreed, through discussion, that each person would respect and uphold the agreement.

After completing the first performance assignment, the class revisited the agreement to see if there were any additional ideas or items that might have arisen from that rehearsal and performance experience. The agreement was revised, agreed to, and then the same reflection was completed after the second performance assignment. This repeated assessment actively reminded students that the agreement was a living document and that their evolving needs were consistently part of the equation in having a community agreement that allowed for everyone's voice to be heard. It gave students the opportunity to speak their needs and have them validated as they grew in the coursework and were partnered with different peers. Scheduling times for reflection on the agreement, as opposed to simply telling students at the beginning of the semester that it could be changed, helped to foster a space where it was understood that what we need today may not be what we need next week or next month and that it is important to delineate space to reflect on that.

As discussed in the chapter on programmatic policy, having universal language for your entire department establishes a consistent baseline of expectation. This can be available on your program's website and can also be standard language included on each course syllabus. Additionally, course-specific syllabus language can contextualize how consent and the commitment to equity and inclusion that underlie it will be applied in each classroom environment. Below are some samples of syllabus language that address these ideas.

Zev Steinrock, University of Illinois Urbana-Champaign (This language is an adaptation from an inclusivity statement originally written by Adam Noble, head of the MFA acting program at the University of Houston.)

Inclusivity:

Every student, regardless of background, ethnicity or identity categories, is a valued member of this ensemble. We all come from different experiences and perspectives, but no one perspective or experience has more value or import than another. Students are encouraged to share their perspective as it is relevant to the course, but no student in this course will be presumed to speak for anything more than their own experience or point of view. Furthermore, in this classroom, you have the right to determine your own identity. You have the right to be called by whatever name you wish, and for that name to be pronounced correctly. You have the right to be referred to by whatever pronoun you wish. You have the right to adjust those things at any point in your education. If there is an aspect of the instruction of this course that results in barriers to your inclusion, or creates a sense of alienation from course content, please contact me privately without fear of reprisal.

(Steinrock 2022a)

Ashleigh Reade, Boston University

I have absolutely zero interest in being a part of an environment, artistic or otherwise, that isn't radically transparent, kind, and rooted in perspective. I want us to look forward to, and enjoy, being together each week. It is my personal belief that voice class is really about listening better, not speaking better. So, let's **listen** with generosity and care, **respond** with generosity and care, and **create** with generosity and care.

(Reade 2022)

Elaine DiFalco Daugherty, Central Michigan University

Consent-based practices in the work:

While physical work may include contact between and among bodies, you and you alone are the keeper of your body. You determine how and when it is used and for what purpose. I will endeavor to foster an environment of active consent that allows each person to speak their boundaries and have them respected. This means that there will be equitable options or alternatives offered for those who may not wish to make physical contact with others. We will discuss consent-based practices in class.

Heather Trommer-Beardslee, Central Michigan University

Touch as a Tool for Correction

As dancers, our body is our instrument, and you, and only you, are in charge of that instrument. Your education is important to me as is prioritizing your bodily autonomy. Physical touch is one of many methods used for making corrections to dance technique. However, you do not have to be touched to receive a good dance education. When I notice that a correction is needed, I will ask if I may touch you, and I will be specific about the type of touch and its purpose. If your answer is no, I will use an alternate, equitable, touchless method. For some people, physical touch works well and for others, it doesn't. Alternatively, if I am using a non-touch method of correction and you would prefer me to use physical touch, please let me know. We feel differently in and about our bodies every day and it is therefore acceptable and expected that your choices about giving or withholding consent to be touched may vary throughout the semester.

Syllabus language that contextualizes consent practices within the specific framework of a given course provides students a glimpse into how you plan to run the space. However, it does not preclude the need for ongoing discussion about and/or facilitation of consent-based practices. Without follow-up, the syllabus note becomes performative and has no traction to be taken at face value by the students. You've got to follow thought with action.

Establishing Boundaries

As stated in her children's book, *Consent for Kids: Boundaries, Respect, and Being in Charge of You*, Rachel Brian writes, "Consent is like being the ruler of your own country. Population: You. Being the ruler of your body means, your body is yours. As a ruler, you get to set your own boundaries. A boundary is a limit" (Brian 2020: 5–8). Although this book was written for young children, the simplicity and directness of this definition are accessible for all readers regardless of age. Open, honest conversations about where our boundaries lie are essential to keeping consent at the center of our work. If we share information in our syllabi, teach from a consent-based perspective, and foster space that allows for continued discussion of consent we're already making great strides. It may take some time and patience for the students to speak up, and more time and more patience for the students to speak their full truth. Keeping in mind that they represent a broad range of learning styles and an even broader range of lived experience, we understand that some students may jump right in and seize the opportunity to be heard while others may linger at the edges to see how it goes for their peers first. If they've only ever known the teacher-as-ruler dynamic, they may need some time to test the waters of this new paradigm and settle into what may be a major shift in their academic world.

We can facilitate students' understanding of what it looks and sounds like to establish boundaries by modeling that behavior for them. Boundaries for teachers? Yes! Who better to model it for them? As Kaja Dunn stated in a 2019 interview, "That seems like a good way to share the work: to acknowledge that we're in this process too. This isn't easy for any of us" (Fairfield 2019: 85). By speaking up for ourselves and creating clear boundaries for our work in educational spaces we not only demonstrate the process for our students but we double-down on our investment in the process by stepping into it even before they do. We need to model that self-care routine to further impress upon our students how vital it is to the longevity of our careers. In our interview with Ann James, she said what we all know to be true:

> We as faculty always try to take on way too damn much. We take on so much that our personal lives suffer, our professional lives suffer, our spiritual lives suffer, because we're just trying to pack a calendar that has no room.

When talking about self-care we've frequently told our students some version of "I'm so good at giving this advice, but not so great at taking it." Now is the time to work to remedy that. As Ann said, the presentation slides about self-care that she shares with students are "a reminder to myself. YOU (talking to myself) seek help when necessary" (James 2022).

Discomfort vs. Fear

Performing arts students are asked to do things that students in more STEM-focused courses aren't. Musicians may be told they need to play with an outwardly clear passion, dancers to move in a way that demonstrates their emotional connection to the story of their movement, stage managers to bear witness to a simulated assault each night. These facets of our work are not traditionally part of daily education and training outside of our spaces; we've never had a pre-med student tell us that their bio-chem professor asked them to be emotionally available in their lab work. For the students who are in our spaces to try something new, there needs to be a standard of care and respect that facilitates their (often new and scary) exploration of what we have to offer. For the students who are in our spaces training to work as performing arts professionals, there needs to be the same care and respect that not only supports their exploration as they grow and develop but that is established as the standard for what they should expect in the profession when they finish their academic career with us. This emotionally heightened work requires students to step out of their established comfort zone and into discomfort which means that we need to establish a trusting space where majors and non-majors alike can engage in a way that is meaningful for them while allowing them to feel supported.

How do we guide students in their discovery of the difference between a firm boundary and the inherent discomfort of trying something they've never tried before? Sterling Hawkins writes,

> As uncomfortable as it is, we don't get a pass from facing the unknown and its harbinger, change. It's an inherent part of life. Most people hear that as bad news. The truth is, on the other side of the unknown are all the results you are looking for. What news could be better than that? When you turn toward discomfort, you will discover a compass leading you to what you want most.
>
> (Hawkins 2022: 4)

In some instances, students will need clear, ongoing discussion about how to investigate their own boundaries and how to learn to discern the sometimes subtle and challenging-to-detect differences between when they are uncomfortable (trying something new, unknown, not threatening), when they are fearful (trying something that threatens their physical or mental safety), and when additional information or support can help move experiences from one category to the other. Laura Rikard, who has been discussing this concept in her classes since 2008 explained,

> Especially in the performing arts, there are certainly going to be times that we are going to be uncomfortable. Where do you get comfortable with Hamlet's uncle killing his father and marrying his mother? The question is how within your boundaries do we tell that story?
>
> (Rikard 2023)

It's important for us to remember that these are our students' journeys and while we may offer guidance and serve as a sounding board for their questions or concerns, it is not our job to tell students where their boundaries lie. In placing value on supporting their autonomy, we accept that the decisions they make about their boundaries are theirs and theirs alone.

One tool for opening this discussion and introducing students to the process of honest self-reflection is *The Discomfort Scale* (see Figure 1). As illustrated in Jessica Steinrock's dissertation, "Intimacy direction: A new role in contemporary theatre making," this diagram illustrates the journey from one's comfort zone into discomfort and the learning that can occur as we move further away from comfort and into new experiences. It also illustrates the edge of the discomfort zone which crosses over into pain or injury and can ultimately lead to trauma if the edge is not observed and respected. This graphic breaks down the complex process and creates access points into thoughtful, productive self-analysis about boundary exploration as an integrated component of education and continued growth (Steinrock 2020).

Another resource for this conversation is Momentum Stage's *Boundary or Comfort Zone* diagram (see Figure 2). Created by the organization's founder, Nicole Perry, this graphic breaks down a range of possible feelings one may have as they navigate new or unfamiliar experiences and work through assessing their needs. In addition to the range in *The Discomfort Scale*, this graphic includes keywords and phrases that can help someone articulate what they are experiencing in the moment. It delineates four markers that categorize experiences as falling within the "confidence zone," the "stretch zone," the "risk zone," and the "boundary zone" as we move from activities that are most comfortable to least comfortable and outside of our boundaries. This exploration allows individuals to examine what they're going through, how they feel about it, how it may potentially make them feel, and then make an informed decision about whether or not to participate in the activity (Perry 2022).

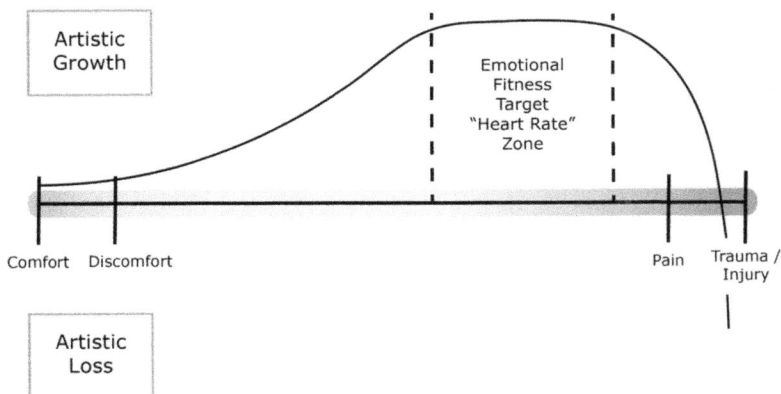

FIGURE 1: The Discomfort Scale as illustrated in Jessica Steinrock's dissertation, "Intimacy direction: A new role in contemporary theatre making." This concept was developed in collaboration with Teri Ciofalo and Zev Steinrock at the University of Illinois.

IS IT A BOUNDARY OR IS IT JUST "OUTSIDE MY COMFORT ZONE"?

These markers might help you determine if something is a boundary for you or is simply uncomfortable. Either way, it is ultimately your decision what material and activities to engage in.

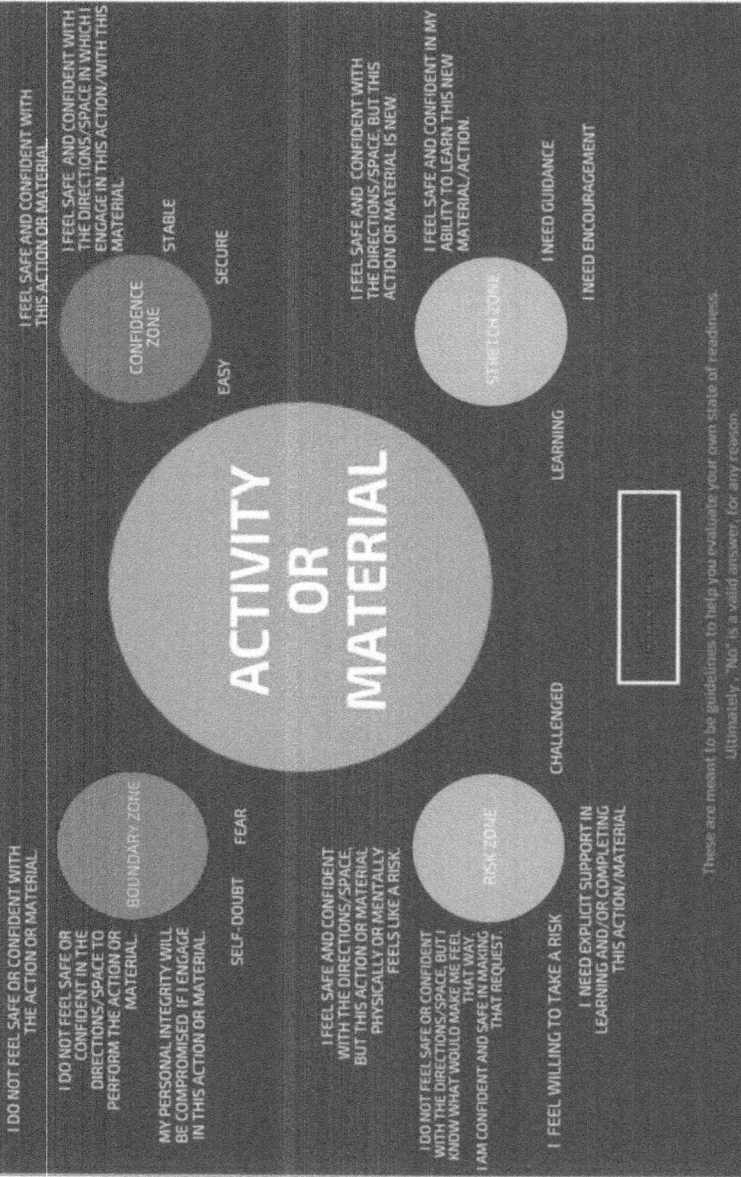

ACTIVITY OR MATERIAL

CONFIDENCE ZONE

STABLE
SECURE
EASY

I FEEL SAFE OR CONFIDENT WITH THE ACTION OR MATERIAL

I FEEL SAFE AND CONFIDENT WITH THE DIRECTIONS/SPACE IN WHICH I ENGAGE IN THIS ACTION/WITH THIS MATERIAL

STRETCH ZONE

LEARNING

I FEEL SAFE AND CONFIDENT WITH THE DIRECTIONS/SPACE, BUT THIS ACTION OR MATERIAL IS NEW

I FEEL SAFE AND CONFIDENT IN MY ABILITY TO LEARN THIS NEW MATERIAL/ACTION.

I NEED GUIDANCE

I NEED ENCOURAGEMENT

BOUNDARY ZONE

FEAR
SELF-DOUBT

I DO NOT FEEL SAFE OR CONFIDENT WITH THE ACTION OR MATERIAL

I DO NOT FEEL SAFE OR CONFIDENT IN THE DIRECTIONS/SPACE TO PERFORM THE ACTION OR MATERIAL.

MY PERSONAL INTEGRITY WILL BE COMPROMISED IF I ENGAGE IN THIS ACTION OR MATERIAL.

RISK ZONE

CHALLENGED

I FEEL SAFE AND CONFIDENT WITH THE DIRECTIONS/SPACE, BUT THIS ACTION OR MATERIAL PHYSICALLY OR MENTALLY FEELS LIKE A RISK.

I DO NOT FEEL SAFE OR CONFIDENT WITH THE DIRECTIONS/SPACE, BUT I KNOW WHAT WOULD MAKE ME FEEL THAT WAY.

I AM CONFIDENT AND SAFE IN MAKING THAT REQUEST.

I FEEL WILLING TO TAKE A RISK

I NEED EXPLICIT SUPPORT IN LEARNING AND/OR COMPLETING THIS ACTION/MATERIAL

These are meant to be guidelines to help you evaluate your own state of readiness. Ultimately, "No" is a valid answer, for any reason.

FIGURE 2: Boundary or comfort zone diagram created by Nicole Perry of Momentum Stage.

The *Yes-to-No Spectrum* (see Figure 3) created by Mia Schachter of Consent Wizardry gets right to the heart of the fact that consent is much more complex than "yes" and "no." If we were to superimpose *The Discomfort Scale* over this graphic, we would clearly see the "yes" line up with the comfort zone section and the "no" line up with the pain/trauma section. Additionally though, this spectrum articulates the nuanced spaces in between those responses and some of the possibilities and potential of what may lie there. It also illustrates a marked shift in the thought process as we move from the "yes" end that internally weighs the possibility of granting consent against personal needs and desires ("What would that feel like?") to the "no" end that weighs it externally against the desired response of others ("What will they think of me?"). This can help clarify where boundaries are by alerting students to being mindful of that shift. Are they making choices based on what is truthfully best for their learning and development, or based on what will be best received by those around them? (Schachter 2022a).

Schachter further explained the thought process by stating that it's important to remember that

we can't avoid doing stuff on the 'no' side. What's crucial there is implementing before, during, and after care so that we move through it consciously and

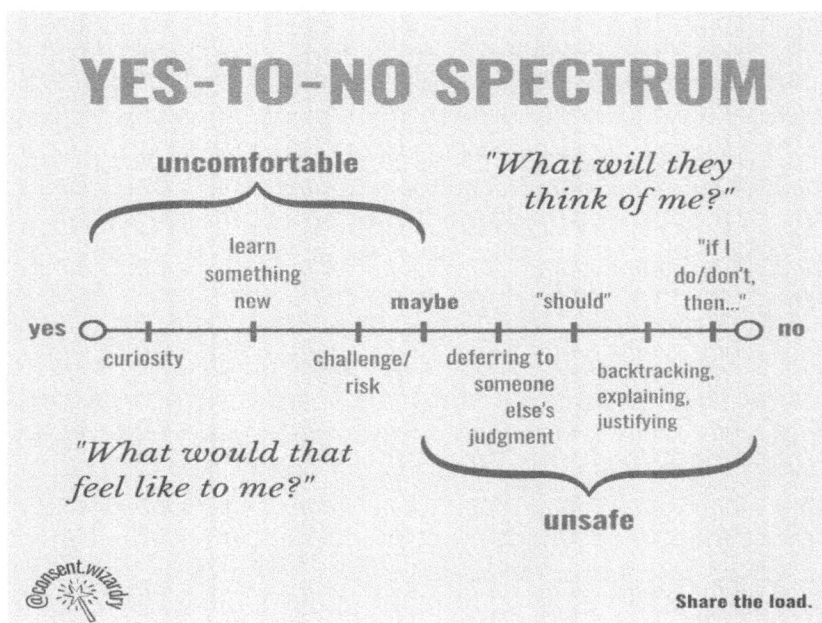

FIGURE 3: Yes-to-no spectrum diagram created by Mia Schachter of Consent Wizardry.

thoughtfully, without denying or trying to convince ourselves that it is in fact something that we want. That would be gaslighting ourselves and our bodies. This requires acknowledging, 'I'm doing something I don't want to do and I'm going to make sure I'm doing it carefully with my care plan in place' as opposed to trying to convince myself, 'This is for my own good,' or otherwise denying my feelings about it.

(Schachter 2022b)

In his work as a technical director at Central Michigan University, Dan Daugherty frequently teaches students who are initially fearful of using power tools that are very loud, or ladders that take them high off the ground, or the intimidating welding process which to a novice, simply looks like melting metal with blinding sparks of light. He lets students know right up front that no one is required to use any of the equipment or undertake any activities that are beyond their personal boundaries. This is for their safety as well as his; forcing a student to use a chop saw or climb a 12-foot ladder against their will is not good for anyone. While he doesn't have a discussion with students about consent perse, he teaches from a consensual perspective. We found this to be the case for many of the educators that we interviewed; they had some practices in place that clearly spoke to an awareness of consent-forward work although they may not have been codified as consent protocols. Universally, the educators we spoke with as part of our research process all had their eyes on the future and the further development of those practices.

Daugherty does not teach with touch as students learn to use tools, hang lights, rig, etc. "I don't do it because I don't find the idea of reaching around someone and holding their hand to be an effective way of teaching" (Daugherty 2022a). He takes an individualized approach in instructing students on how to safely handle whatever they're ready to handle. Some students enter the shop for the first time eager to get their hands on new equipment and to do the scary thing right in the moment. Other students need to be introduced to the activity/equipment, given some time to process it (maybe until the next class, maybe until next week), and then find their way to being open to trying it. Still others are introduced, given time to process, and don't ever find themselves in a space where the activity is within their boundaries.

This is reflective of how Zev Steinrock described the accommodation of different learning styles in his stage combat class at University of Illinois. It's about acknowledging the difference between

the actor who, in order to actually learn the thing they have to see someone do it. Or in order to actually learn the thing, they need to see someone do it and talk about what they're doing while they're doing it. Or in order to actually learn the thing, none of that was helpful. They just need enough [information and instruction] to kind of try it and then begin to learn when they actually start doing the thing. Or some of them will try in the room and won't actually learn it until they go to sleep that night and rest on it and come back the next day.

(Steinrock 2022b)

Being able to do the thing at the moment is not what's crucial, learning how to learn it is.

To further encourage the expansion of the comfort zone in an incremental manner, Daugherty offers in-between options for students to try out. If someone is unable to say yes to climbing a 12-foot ladder they can try a smaller stepladder first. Once they're comfortable with that, there is a 4-foot ladder option. Perhaps that's where they stop, perhaps they're eventually interested in attempting the 12-foot ladder. The person above the stage walking the grid may have initially been fearful of that work. If they're forced to try, they're much more likely to resist and withdraw. If they're in charge of their learning, they're more likely to engage and attempt at their own pace.

Daugherty believes that this is the most effective manner of instruction. It keeps students in the driver's seat as they test new and potentially scary tasks. If they're afforded a genuine opportunity to opt out and then re-engage when prepared to do so, they have agency over that reengagement. Additionally, he believes that if we teach them that they have to do something in order to work professionally (in the case of his students, as technical theatre practitioners) it provides an inaccurately narrow perception of the profession.

When we say "well, this is what it takes to be a professional," it is inherently exclusionary because you're talking about one version of a professional in the industry. When we say we're training them so that they know what it means to be in the profession, part of that has to be an acknowledgement of the range of the profession.

(Daugherty 2022b)

Both Daugherty's and Steinrock's approaches reflect the difference between how students may have been treated and taught in the past vs. how we want to treat them moving forward. When we employ a narrow mindset and insist on a singular process for all learners, we are more likely to create an environment that is *exclusive* rather than *inclusive*. We want to open up space for them and to show them that there is a place for them in the art.

REFERENCES

Bain, K. (2004), *What the Best College Teachers Do*, Cambridge, MA: Harvard University Press.

Bones, C. D. W. (2022), interviewed by E. Daugherty and H. Trommer-Beardslee, Online 23 May 2022.

Brian, R. (2020), *Consent (For Kids!): Boundaries, Respect, and Being in Charge of You*, Boston, MA: Little Brown Books, pp. 5–8.

Daugherty, D. (2022a), interviewed by E. Daugherty and H. Trommer-Beardslee, Central Michigan University, 20 May 2022.

Daugherty, D. (2022b), interviewed by E. Daugherty, Blaze Pizza, Mount Pleasant, MI on 27 May 2022.

Fairfield, J. B., Sina, T., Rikard, L. and Dunn, K. (2019), "Intimacy choreography and culture change: An interview with leaders in the field," *Journal of Dramatic Theory and Criticism*, 34:1, pp. 77–85.

Hawkins, S. (2022), *Hunting Discomfort: How to Get Results in Life and Business No Matter What*, Los Angeles, CA: Wonderwell, p. 4.

James, A. (2022), interviewed by E. Daugherty and H. Trommer-Beardslee, Online 24 May 2022.

Perry, N. (2022), personal communication, 4 May 2022.

Reade, A. (2022), personal communication, 31 May 2022.

Rikard, L. (2023), interviewed by E. Daugherty and H. Trommer-Beardslee, Online 9 June 2023.

Schachter, M. (2022a), personal communication, 5 August 2022.

Schachter, M. (2022b), personal communication, 5 August 2022.

Steinrock, J. (2020), *Intimacy Direction: A New Role in Contemporary Theatre Making*, Urbana, IL: University of Illinois Urbana-Champaign, pp. 167–74.

Steinrock, Z. (2022a), personal communication, 26 May 2022.

Steinrock, Z. (2022b), interviewed by E. Daugherty and H. Trommer-Beardslee, Online 26 May 2022.

4

Production Facilitation

In performing arts education, production work is a practical extension of the classroom. It affords students the opportunity to take the skills they've been developing in their coursework and apply them in an experiential learning-based setting. While the structures for learning may be different, it only makes sense that the consent practices that we establish in the classroom should be translated to the production environment and the processes surrounding it.

Before we even enter the rehearsal space, there has likely been an audition for those involved. Information provided to students before auditioning for particular shows and roles allows each person to make an informed decision about whether or not they should audition or participate. Audition disclosures include information about expectations for performers based on what the script requires and what the director/choreographer, etc. expects from each participant. Chelsea Pace writes,

> This process creates opportunities for actors to state their boundaries and ask clarifying questions about the demands of a role. Out of a desire to be cast, actors may intentionally or unintentionally misrepresent their boundaries. There is no perfect system, and while the Audition Disclosure process isn't perfect, it creates the most opportunities for consent in casting.
>
> (Pace 2020: 104)

The disclosure can vary greatly from show to show and is most useful when it includes as much detail as is available at the time of posting. For theatrical and dance productions, the audition disclosure may include an action breakdown that details the expectations for each individual role.

The following breakdown for Elaine's auditions for *Dancing at Lughnasa* (see Box 4) covers several details that may be challenging for student performers. Several of the characters sing and dance in the show but aren't necessarily brilliant at either. There is partnered dancing requiring close contact between actors as well

45

CHARACTER	ACTION
CHRIS	partnered dancing with GERRY
	kissed by GERRY (no mouth-to-mouth contact)
MAGGIE	partnered dancing with GERRY
	sings (doesn't have to be a singer)
AGNES	fastest knitter in Ballybeg
	partnered dancing with GERRY
	kissed by GERRY on the hand and/or forehead
ROSE	knitter
	sings (doesn't have to be a singer)
MUNDY SISTERS	dance together with hand holding, arm linking, embracing
	Donegal dialects
MICHAEL	Donegal dialects
JACK	scarcely a trace of Irish dialect
	dances-shuffles and sings (not a singer or dancer)
GERRY	partnerd dancing with CHRIS
	partnered dancing with AGNES
	partnered dancing with MAGGIE
	kisses CHRIS (no mouth-to-mouth contact)
	kisses AGNES on the hand and/or forehead
	Welsh dialect
	sings (doesn't have to be a singer)

Box 4: Action breakdown created by Elaine DiFalco Daugherty for *Dancing at Lughnasa.*

as some kissing. Additionally, there is some very challenging dialect work for the entire cast, and at least one of the actors needs to be able to knit convincingly enough to be seen as "the fastest knitter in Ballybeg" in a small black box space with the audience only inches away. Any one of these requirements may be a deal breaker for an actor considering auditioning for the show.

You can see in the following example that specifics have been included about the physical requirements. These are separated by character and, where possible, are specific to who initiates and who receives an action. Chris is "kissed by GERRY (no mouth-to-mouth contact)." The character of Maggie "sings (doesn't have to be a singer)." Gerry is partnered with three different women to dance over the course of the show. These descriptions clarify details of expectations and allow students to make informed decisions about whether or not their boundaries will allow for them to be successful in a potential role.

ANNIE	X	assists in dressing and undressing of MRS. DALDRY
	X	assists in dressing and undressing of LEO
	X	observes all of DR. GIVINGS' simulated vibrator treatments
	31	simulates manual stimulation of MRS. DALDRY who simulates ejaculation
	74	simulates administering vibrator treatment on MRS. DALDRY who simulates loud orgasm
	75	engages in "weirdly compromised post-coital" position with MRS. DALDRY
	78	kisses MRS. DALDRY on the mouth

Box 5: Action breakdown excerpt created by Elaine DiFalco Daugherty for *In the Next Room, or the vibrator play.*

Audition disclosures may also include information about heightened language, various stages of required undress and/or nudity, and any other pertinent information that may influence someone's decision to participate. If there are non-negotiable actions (i.e., a character has to fire a prop gun), that should be marked as such on the breakdown. When serving as the intimacy director for *In the Next Room or the vibrator play*, Elaine created an action breakdown which was posted with the audition notice (see Box 5). The sample section shows the anticipated actions for the character of Annie. The second column is page numbers of actions or "x" denoting that it occurs several times throughout the script. Note the clear distinction between actions that would be completed vs. actions that would be simulated. No actor needs to give another actor an actual treatment—that's simulated through specific choreography that mimics and/or masks and appears to be truthful administration of the treatment. However, the actor playing Annie does assist in the dressing and undressing of other characters and needs to be aware of that requirement. She also bears witness to each of Dr Givings' treatments and so watches as other characters appear to orgasm.

When creating disclosure documents, think about what you'd want to know about a character you may have to play before agreeing to play the role. Does the show deal with a particular topic or set of ideas/ideals that may be outside of your boundaries? Does the character appear in a bathing suit? Does the character iterate derogatory language? If you'd want to know about it ahead of time, include it in the document; better to over-disclose than under-disclose. Keep in mind that even if a character does not engage in a particular action, they may be required to witness the action (a sexual assault, for instance)—include that information as well.

Dance audition disclosures can also help potential auditionees make decisions about their boundaries. The chart (see Box 6) is based on a dance concert with

Dance Company Auditions

Dance Piece	Physical Requirements
Ballet	pas de deux: partner dancing with lifts that will include multiple points of physical contact
Modern	some partner contact with no weight sharing
Hip-hop	contact between hands/arms/shoulders of dancers
Tap	contact between hands/arms/shoulders of dancers
Ballet #2	some partner contact with no weight sharing
Modern # 2	partner work with moments of weight share at several contact points
Irish Step	contact between hands/arms/shoulders/waists of dancers
Tap #2	no contact
Jazz	no contact

Box 6: Action breakdown for a dance company concert.

curated pieces that have already been choreographed. It shows the requirements for each piece and clarifies what the choreographers have in mind for the dancers they cast. Even if the piece has not been fully choreographed, it is helpful to disclose if the choreographer plans physical contact, weight share, or will be using thematic content that may be difficult.

A dance company audition disclosure could also include a third column with information about the story of each dance to further clarify the storytelling content in addition to the physical requirements. This will be dependent on the story or thematic content that each choreographer is intending to portray. If the dance relies on heightened content, including that information in a disclosure prior to the audition would be appropriate.

These disclosures are supported by audition applications that include questions reflective of this information. Perhaps in the case of the dance concert, the application asks dancers to check which dances they are interested in being considered for, or to cross out any that they are not willing to be part of. Theatre auditions can do the same with audition sheets that ask which roles the actor would like to be considered for. The audition sheet for *In the Next Room* ... included a section with the statement "I have read both the script and the action breakdown and am interested in auditioning for the following roles:" This allowed students to mark their choices for consideration based on their boundaries without having to discuss or justify those choices.

This same disclosure process can be used for musicians who will comprise the pit orchestra for a musical or individual musicians providing live scoring for a play. Traditionally, orchestras work independently of the staging of the show until sitzprobe when musicians and singers finally hear each other's work and/or wandelprobe when the orchestra may first see some of the staging. Although the musicians are watching their scores and the conductor, there are any number of instances when one or more musicians may not be playing a part of a song and end up watching the action on stage. If their work will require them to witness violence or nudity or other actions that are outside of their boundaries, they should be made aware of those aspects of the show before agreeing to participate. This holds true for when musicians are on stage as an integrated part of the action of the show (e.g., a structure like *Hadestown*), when the orchestra needs to take musical cues off of the action in the show, when a band is located on the stage in full view of the audience, or when individual musicians are scoring dance and scene work live.

Backstage and Offstage Consent Practices

These foundational practices carry over into all spaces and opportunities, including non-performance areas. This means creating a process and timeline for how and when the production team (both students and additional staff and faculty) are provided disclosure information before agreeing to work as crew on the production. To simplify, the same disclosures that are used for the audition process can be made available for potential production team members to review before signing on. In an academic setting, this is especially important if the production work is being used as a studio or independent study credit. Students need to know what they're committing to before consenting to tie it to an academic requirement.

Implementing consent practices for offstage work is no different than for onstage work. All of the same basic principles apply in all places. For instance, a student learning to be a sound technician needs to be informed that it involves physical contact with others and that the contact is generally on and around the face and hair and/or down the back and under clothing. As they are preparing to do the actual work of micing an actor, there needs to be communication before any contact is made. In scheduling rehearsal time, this could be done as an overview by the sound op for the entire cast before individuals are actually mic'd. A simple introduction can go a long way, so introduce yourself, your pronouns, and your role in the work before explaining the logistics. Then talk the performer(s) through the process of securing microphones. Following is an outline of how a sample conversation might go. Keep in mind that the process is in place to acknowledge and uphold boundaries for both parties involved.

- Introductions
- Explanation of the process (parts, locations, steps to completion)
- Do you have any questions?
- Are you ready to be mic'd?
- Speak through the steps

  Technician: "The belt pack needs to be secured around your waist. Would you prefer I secure it or that you secure it and then I check it?"

  Actor: "It doesn't matter to me."

  Technician: "Then I'd prefer that you secure it and I check it afterwards."

Think of the process of securing the mic as choreography so that it happens the same way every time. When possible, minimize contact during the process and then wrap up by checking in to ensure that the secured mic does not interfere with costume/wig/movement, etc. Removal at the end of the rehearsal or show can happen in reverse fashion.

These same principles can be applied to costuming as the wardrobe crew prepares for any dressing or undressing that necessitates assistance. Daugherty et al. state the following in their article, "Offstage intimacy: Best practices for navigating the intimacy of costuming,"

> as with any part of running a show, quick changes must be rehearsed and choreographed with the actor, wardrobe attendant, and the wardrobe supervisor or designer. First, provide an opportunity for introduction and exchange of consent. Similar to choreographed intimacy, costume changes should be crafted as a series of physical actions that are specific and repeatable. Identify which costume pieces are coming off and which are going on and establish choreography for the change. Identify who is responsible for handling each piece of clothing, accessories, and even the process of fastening and securing the garment. These changes should be worked through slowly at first to allow for the planning of the mechanics of the change and incorporating any necessary adjustments. Once the changes can be done accurately, speed can be increased.
>
> (Daugherty 2020: 214)

One of the most eye-opening interviews we conducted was with Chels Morgan who is the only person we spoke with who has experience working as a circus aerial rigger. For those unfamiliar, in circus work, aerial riggers safely hang, set, and secure performers' apparatuses in preparation for their act. In some cases, they assist the aerialist during their act, flying them either by manual pulley system or via a motorized zip lift, called a winch, that they operate with a handheld pendant. In our discussion with Chels, they talked about how the performer's apparatus is treated as an extension of the performer.

It's like touching your body, so I'm not gonna touch it in a way that is uncomfortable for you. How do you want me to check it? Do you want me to check it? Do you want to do it? How does this work? So that's a huge thing: consent around their apparatus as a part of their body.

They went on to talk about the work of maintaining the conversation non-verbally during the act.

At any point I could ram this joystick up and take you up. So what sort of nonverbal check-ins do we have? What if something goes wrong and you're in pain? How do you tell me without alerting the entire audience? It's almost like partnering in dance. The rigger operating the apparatus is one dancer and the performer is the other. So, I have to ask for consent in the same way that partners in dance would ask for consent. There's a lot that goes into that, and it's a really strong trust-based relationship.

(Morgan 2022)

Before this conversation, we hadn't thought about the work of circus performers as part of our scope, but the comparison to the way consent communication functions between partnered dancers opened up a little window in our thought processes. Additionally, the idea of apparatus and the way it is treated as an extension of the performer got us thinking about parallels to the etiquette surrounding how we treat musicians' instruments. Our thoughts were confirmed when Andrée Martin told us that in early lessons instrumentalists are taught to not touch other people's instruments and that she works in a way that keeps her hands off her students' flutes. In the past, she may have put her hand under the drooping end of a flute to correct parallel alignment with the player's lip but now she simply places a pencil into the end of the flute. If their alignment slips the pencil slides out onto the floor and the student knows to correct the alignment. They may end up picking up the pencil many times over the course of a lesson, but it certainly is an effective tool for heightening alignment awareness while upholding the boundary and modeling the behavior of not handling another person's instrument (Martin 2022).

Establishing Expectations and Guidelines

In the same manner that course-specific language in a syllabus provides context, so can a set of guidelines built intentionally for an individual show. Universal protocols may already be established for general behavioral expectations in your program's productions, but having additional standards in place for how your specific show will be handled can further support your students.

The first rehearsal is the time to establish how everyone will engage with the work. This engagement may be different for each individual depending on varying needs, backgrounds, and experiences. Everyone will bring something different that could influence how they interact, what they offer, and what they may need during the production process. This is a great opportunity to facilitate the creation of a community agreement (this process is outlined in Chapter Three), or to review the standards already in place for your program. What's important is for the production facilitator(s) to set the tone for how the group will move forward together in the collaborative process and to model that behavior right from the get go. Offer students an opportunity to ask questions and let them know that the opportunity to ask questions doesn't end there, but will be available throughout the process. Remind them of the importance of communication and introduce whatever chain of communication has been established for the production. If you've made an action breakdown available prior to auditions, your students already know that you are placing value on their autonomy in the process, but an additional outline of rehearsal expectations may be beneficial. The following is an excerpt from CMU's Rehearsal Process Guidelines and Expectations for Cast and Crew from a production of *Indecent* by Paula Vogel (see Box 7).

If there is an intimacy director for the production, set aside some time in the first rehearsal to allow that person to introduce themself and speak about the process of how heightened material will be handled. If there isn't an intimacy director on the production team, that information can still be conveyed through the director who will be handling the discussion and choreography of that material.

If your program currently has a face mask policy in place, be sure to discuss the details of the policy and if/when masks may be removed as technical rehearsals approach. Discuss best practices for hygiene to keep individuals and the group as a whole as healthy as possible. If there is no masking mandate, allow space to discuss how the group feels about masking as a precaution. Let students know that if wearing a mask will allow them greater ease and therefore allow them to do better work in the rehearsal space, that they should wear a mask until they're ready to remove it or up until the scheduled date when all masks will be removed for technical rehearsals.

No matter the needs of a specific production and the needs of the individual people involved in creating it, the expectations for how those needs will be met must be centered on creating a practical learning environment that prioritizes consent and autonomy.

The rehearsal room is a space to safely experiment and explore material with mutual focus and consideration.This requires us to step outside of our comfort zones and trust each other to work respectfully and thoughtfully in service of the text. It is each of our responsibilities, individually and collectively, to foster a culture of continuous consent and open communication. This inherently includes the expectations of equitable treatment, privacy, and encouragement. To that end, the following information is provided as a framework for the process of developing the show together.

1. Consent
Our rehearsal process is consent-based; this is a commitment made by the Department of Theatre and Dance and by each of the members of the faculty and staff. Regardless of who is running the room in a given rehearsal, you are entitled to work in a space that respects you as an individual and upholds your boundaries and needs.

2. Choreography
As we work on choreography, (intimacy, dance, and fight) our goal is to create specific, repeatable action that focuses the text and creates purposeful storytelling while respecting individual boundaries. This may begin as structured improvisation or pre-built choreography; either way, direction will be given in terms of physical movement using desexualized language that refers to the action.

3. Accountability
As an actor, you will never be in the room with only one other person working on intimate choreography. There will always be at least one faculty member and a member of the stage management team present. Outside of rehearsal you should not rehearse the intimate physicality of the show with only your scene partner; you should always have at least one other trusted person present.

4. The Button*
Working on this material may be physically and/or emotionally strenuous. During rehearsals, please use the word "button" to indicate that you need a momentary break. This word is offered as a way to gently pause if
    --you need to clarify direction/choreography
    --you need a moment to process your personal response to something
    --you need to stop physical contact because it crosses your personal boundaries
    --you feel that the choreography is not being followed and/or that liberties are
    being taken that expand or alter the material
*The Button was created by Theatrical Intimacy Education.

5. Concern Resolution
Should you experience an incident during the rehearsal period that you feel is a breach of consent and/or respect, the first course of action is to speak up in the moment. If for some reason you do not feel comfortable doing so, you have several options for resolution outlined in the chart below. (This would be followed by a chain of communication appropriate for your program.)

Box 7: Excerpt from Rehearsal Process Guidelines and Expectations created by Elaine DiFalco Daugherty.

REFERENCES

Daugherty, E., Hertzberg, D. and Wagner, D. (2020), "Offstage intimacy: Best practices for navigating the intimacy of costuming," *Theatre Topics*, 30:3, pp. 211–16.

Martin, A. (2022), interviewed by E. Daugherty and H. Trommer-Beardslee, Online 11 August 2022.

Morgan, C. (2022), interviewed by E. Daugherty and H. Trommer-Beardslee, Online 31 May 2022.

Pace, C. and Rikard, L. (2020), *Staging Sex: Best Practices, Tools, and Techniques for Theatrical Intimacy*, New York, NY: Routledge, p. 104.

5

Activities and Strategies for Facilitating Consent Practices

So, what now? You may know that you want to work to create a consent-forward classroom or rehearsal space, but how do you get started? The good news is that the starting is already taking place. You're doing it. The talking about it—the thinking about it and continuing to roll it over in your mind—the reading about it—that is the starting.

The following is a collection of activities and strategies that we gathered during our journey of talking to educators about consent-forward practices. This is the stuff that people are currently doing to prioritize body autonomy in their classrooms. When we set out to answer the question, What are people doing right now?, this is what we discovered. This is the *what*.

We would like to take this opportunity to gently step back and remember Laura Rikard's idea of an "offering" (Rikard 2022) that is used in the introduction of this book. This chapter is a selection of ideas for you to try, modify, or be inspired by to completely invent a new exercise that will work best for you and your students. (If you do that, please share it with us. We would love to hear what you are doing and what is working for you.) We don't imagine that every offering will be the right fit for every classroom. There is no particular order for how or when to use these, so to get started, try one thing. Choose the exercise that you think will work best in your educational setting. As you continue to experiment and modify as needed along the way, you will likely develop a collection of activities that are your go-to tools. You will likely find that different educational circumstances will call for varying activities as is typically the case in all pedagogical endeavors.

An Offering of Activities

Since we just included a reminder of Laura Rikard's idea of an offering, the first activity we are going to offer is one that Laura highly recommended during our interview with her.

Simon Says (with a Twist) (Pace 2020a: 19–20)

This is an activity developed by Theatrical Intimacy Education that can be found in Chelsea Pace's book, *Staging Sex: Best Practices, Tools, and Techniques for Staging Theatrical Intimacy*.

The game starts like any other game of Simon Says. The player who is chosen to play the role of Simon calls out commands.

"Simon says touch your right hand to your head!"

"Simon says put your hands on your hips!"

If "Simon Says" is included in the command, the players need to act on the command, if not, they don't.

Play a few rounds in this traditional way and then add the twist.

Twist One: This time, participants have the option to say "No." when Simon gives a command, even when Simon states, "Simon Says." At any given time, a participant may choose not to do the action, stand still, and say "No."

In this portion of the activity description, Pace suggests the following after playing with the "No" option:

> ask the participants how it felt to say "no" to the person in charge. They may say it felt uncomfortable at first, or it may have made them feel powerful. Some might observe that after they say no, nothing bad happened, which is, of course, the whole point.

Twist Two: Continue playing and this time add a third response option for when Simon gives a command:

Option 1: Do the action as commanded.
Option 2: Say "no" and do not do the action.
Option 3: Say "Button!"

Important note: "Button" is the word used by Theatrical Intimacy Education, to "indicate that the action needs to pause for a moment. Pauses might be to ask a question, clear something up, shake something out, or even to avoid sneezing into someone's face" (Pace 2020b: 17).

If the participant says, "Button," they need to then add an alternative option. For example, "Instead of touching my hand to my forehead, I would like to touch my hand to my nose."

In an e-mail conversation with Pace on June 27, 2023, she added the following information for practitioners leading this exercise:

> One additional parameter that I have been introducing at the beginning of the exercise is offering all participants a general sense of the scope of the types of asks I will

be making. I list a few examples and I make it clear that the purpose of this game and the types of things I'm going to be asking is not to shock them. Sometimes, participants will refrain from saying no in anticipation of me making a "big" ask and that distracts them from the ask in the present.

(Pace 2023)

The Boundary Picnic

This is a variation on I'm Going on a Picnic. In this exercise, participants stand in a circle and speak one at a time in sequence around the circle. One person starts with "I'm (name #1) and one of my boundaries is my right shoulder (or whatever their boundary is)." The person next to them says, "I'm (name #2) and one of my boundaries is my chest and (name #1)'s boundary is her right shoulder." The next person says, "I'm (name #3) and my boundary is my stomach and (name #2)'s boundary is their chest and (name #1)'s boundary is their right shoulder." This continues around the entire circle until returning to the first participant who repeats the entire list of names and boundaries.

The purpose of this activity is to encourage active listening, practice addressing one's own boundaries, and to respect the boundaries of others through accurate acknowledgment. It can be used to share physical boundaries, material boundaries ("my boundary is uttering racial slurs"), or even observational boundaries ("my boundary is witnessing someone undressing someone else"). For this activity to work in a classroom, students do not necessarily need to voice boundaries that actually exist. It can be more about the practice of voicing boundaries and acknowledging the boundaries of others. In the rehearsal space, it can work with a cast as they are introduced to boundary exercises. In this case, it would be more useful for articulating actual boundaries. In either case, you could also modify it to be a completely non-verbal exercise in which participants use their hands to show a physical boundary and each person mimics that physically.

Self-Practice—What We Allow Others to See (and Hear) (Finley 2023a)

Rachel Finley, a theatre professor at Arizona State University, developed the following activity in order to allow her students to engage in consent-forward practices on themselves before working with others. She starts by inviting participants to begin by walking through and enjoying the space. "When you find a space you like, hang out there." Each student finds a space and settles in. Rachel then invites participants to touch their body in every place that they are consenting to having other people witness them touching. The witnessing is one of the components of consent that is sometimes forgotten in rehearsal and yet is very important in the performing arts where we create experiences designed for audiences to witness. It's not just about what you are doing; it is also about what you are allowing others to watch you do.

Rachel conducts a variation of this exercise in which participants experiment with creating sound in front of others. In our interview with her, she reminded us that voice vibrates through the body and therefore creating sound is also an action that must be consented to. What sounds are we willing to let others hear us make?

Only No

There are several versions of this game that have been modified and used by prominent consent-forward organizations. The following is one of Elaine's modifications. She first encountered a version of this activity as "May I" at a Theatrical Intimacy Education workshop in Salt Lake City (Pace 2019). This particular version focuses on flipping the script from "yes" being the expected and acceptable answer, to "no" being the only expected and acceptable answer.

Have the participants form a circle and ask for a volunteer to begin. Person #1 crosses the circle and stands about an arm's length in front of someone else. Seeking eye contact, Person #1 asks Person #2 , "May I touch your shoulder?" Person #2 always responds with "No." Person #1 and Person #2 swap places and Person #2 crosses to someone else to ask the same question. The only response to the question is "no."

As the game progresses, participants may be given the option to provide a counteroffer to the first question. So, rather than saying "no," Person #2 may respond "No, but you may touch the back of my left hand." If Person #2 chooses this option, Person #1 responds with "no" and they swap places. In this version, "yes" isn't even an option for response.

In following this Only No script, each participant walks across the circle knowing they are going to receive a "no" and asks the question knowing they are going to receive a "no." This allows for preparation and processing time to normalize how to receive that response with grace rather than resistance. Additionally, each participant only answers "no" which allows them to practice delivering "no" in a low-stakes environment where there are no repercussions for that answer. The option to add the counteroffer provides an opportunity to practice the offering of a Plan B when the Plan A presented does not fit within personal boundaries.

Past facilitations of this exercise have elicited responses from participants that have included a discussion of the stress of the internal monologue that occurs as Person #1 crosses the circle. Interestingly, the action of crossing the circle was often more nerve-wracking than the giving and receiving of the actual "no." The tension in that anticipation has led to comments about how it might be better to communicate in a direct manner rather than hesitating and allowing for additional time to overthink the decision to ask for what you need.

Beyond Yes and No

This exercise can be facilitated as an exploration of the spectrum of communication with small groups in a classroom environment and/or as a means to discuss how we actually communicate our needs or boundaries in rehearsal spaces with our scene partners. The work here is to learn about the ways we and others might convey that we need time to consider an offer before consenting. This exercise lives in the space between "yes" and "no" on Mia Schachter's Yes-to-No Spectrum.

If working with a small group in a class, we might put eight people in a circle and have them go around one at a time and show the group a way that someone might communicate hesitation. As with The Boundary Picnic, the classroom environment is an exploratory space for learning how to articulate these things, so students don't necessarily have to use only their own physical responses in the exercise. It's good practice to both show their action and perhaps show what they've seen in others. The lead-in phrase can be as simple as, "If I think something might breach my boundaries I might _____." In that blank, they can show the group what might show up in their body as resistance in a moment when they aren't ready/able, etc. to say "yes" or "no." Once they've completed the action and held it for a moment, the facilitator of the group can ask for someone to state the physical response that occurred to ensure understanding and then the exercise moves to the next person. So, perhaps Person #1 states the phrase and fills that blank by tightly pursing their lips together. After a moment of holding the action, the teacher asks for someone to name the response. A volunteer from the group names it and then the next person takes a turn.

If working in a rehearsal setting, scene partners could face each other and alternate that showing and telling. When there are only two people participating, the exercise could move forward without the lead-in phrase after the first exchange and become a sort of tennis match of shared physicality. When they take the time to explore and share these non-verbals, they can establish a somatic vocabulary that goes beyond language and supports deeper understanding of how they function in the moment as they are working.

Practicing Exit Strategies (Steinrock 2022)

Jessica Steinrock, CEO of Intimacy Directors and Coordinators, acknowledges that mistakes will happen. Even with consent protocols in place, people will accidentally cross boundaries. Additionally, participants may realize that a boundary has been crossed that they did not initially address, because they did not know it existed until the moment in which they felt uncomfortable. Jessica leads students in practicing exit strategies in her classes so that students can learn how to step out of difficult situations in a low-stakes environment. This allows them to build the skill set while nothing is at risk so that the skill is in place when needed. Whether it be a distinct turn away, a hand up, or a hand to one's own chest, each participant develops an exit strategy signal that is practiced with the class so that it is in their body for when it is needed. Then this practice continues through the duration of the semester or run of the class to keep it in the body so that it is readily accessible when needed.

The Comfort Play (Quinnett 2022)

This activity for modeling honest communication, empathy, and respect of personal boundaries was developed by Kelly Quinnett, head of acting at the University of Idaho. She explains,

> People aren't typically taught how to be in communication with each other—a real connected circular communication. We are usually taught to communicate in ways that are appropriate or perceived to be good. We are taught to conform. I was curious how to get people to experience what it is like to be held in someone's presence.
> (Quinnett 2022)

After leading this exercise on its own for many years, Kelly now pairs it with TIE's boundary exercise. This way, the activity follows a conversation in which participants name their personal boundaries and those boundaries are upheld throughout the action of the play. A facilitator then leads the pairs through a three-act play in which partners are A & B:

> Act 1: A's super objective is to give comfort to B because they are wired to do so. B's super objective is to receive comfort from A because they are wired to do so.
> Act 2: A & B switch as giver and receiver.
> Act 3: A & B take on both super objectives and must give and receive comfort because they are wired to do so.

The giving of comfort can take many forms depending on the boundaries previously set by both involved participants. It could be prolonged continuous eye contact, hand holding, an embrace, or countless other methods, as long as it meets the boundary parameters set by both parties. This can be tricky and therefore teaches active listening and engagement in creating practices that work for everyone involved even when the answer is not simple.

As a facilitator of this exercise, be careful not to rush through the acts. Give time for the participants to work through the process and have the opportunity to see and be seen by their partner. Anywhere between five and ten minutes per act will provide space for partners to truly witness each other and provide comfort that is specific to each individual.

The Game (Joynt Sandberg 2022a)

This is an activity that was shared with us by Liz Joynt Sandberg, Head of Comedy Arts at The Theatre School at DePaul University. She modified it from an activity used by The Second City Training Center. In the way that Liz currently uses it, this activity facilitates an understanding of participant power, autonomy, the teacher as a collaborator, and the importance of making mistakes in order to learn what doesn't work.

Begin the game by having the students gather in a group; this typically will instinctually end up being a circle. Tell everyone that you're going to play a game but you won't be telling them the rules of the game. You will let them know when they do something that is outside of the way the game is played. The teacher facilitates the start of the game by clapping their hands and then pointing to a person in the group while making eye contact with them. (That's it. The game has begun.) At this point, the teacher waits for the students to play the game; whatever happens, happens. The students are in charge.

The students will have questions and questions are great! Students should absolutely be encouraged to ask themselves questions during the game, answer their own questions, and then implement the answers in their work during the game. Students should trust that their answers are true. The goal is to get students experimenting with what works and what doesn't and communicating as they go. They are in control, and figuring that out is a major point of the game.

After playing for a bit and guiding the students only by telling them when they've done something outside of the way the game is played, pause the game and ask if anyone can say with certainty that they know the rules of the game and can play it correctly. Anyone who says "yes" is asked to form an inner circle and to teach the outer circle the rules by continuing to play the game.

The game is chaotic and can take on an infinite number of forms because the students develop it as they go. It can also be extremely frustrating for students because they are not provided with all the information that they feel they need to be successful.

The game is played until the students "win," and there are only two ways to win (but they don't know the ways to win until they have won):

1. Every person playing the game decides that they understand the rules of the game and steps into the inner circle.
2. The students mutiny and just stop. They could decide to not play.

Thinking back to previous times that she has used this activity in class, Liz explains,

I have had students be frustrated and want to quit and I've responded, "Ok. That feels like information. If you want to quit, then quit." There's lots of stuff that shows up. The simple reality is that students can stop whenever they want. And actually, that's a way to win. The students decide how to complete the assignment and how to demonstrate what they've learned. They are often so furious once they discover that. The Game is unmitigated chaos. It's wild—especially when we realize what is actually at the core. It is an ideological application of true agency in action.

Betty Martin's Three Activity Suggestions (Martin 2023)

In our interview with Betty Martin, she provided us with several suggestions for activities (original creators unknown) that she has adapted over the years to focus on consent. All three of the activity offerings from Martin are detailed here:

1. Yes/No Walk and Talk
   This activity starts with a group of people walking through the space—no set patterns, just walking. After walking and exploring the space, stop the entire group, and each individual says the word no. They can say it a few different times, altering the way they say it each time. (They aren't saying no to anything in particular.) Repeat the walking and stopping to say no a few times.

   After this goes on for a few minutes, have the group stop and talk about what this felt like in their body. How did it feel to say no? Describe the physical sensations that were felt as a result of saying no.

   Then, repeat the same activity, but this time in the pauses, say the word yes. Notice what it feels like in the body to say yes and talk about it as a group.

   Continue walking around the room and when you find yourself face to face with another person, notice in your body whether you are a yes to this person or a no. Don't convey the answer. Just notice it in your body. Stay near that person for half a minute and then move on to someone else. Notice the physical sensations that give you information about yes and no.

   Through this activity, participants learn to tune into the information that their body provides itself and to use that information to assess their needs.

   A final step in the activity is to pair up and have a yes/no conversation. Again, these aren't answers to any question in particular, just words for the purpose of noticing the sensations that are caused by saying them. In this conversation, participants stand face to face saying yes or no in response to each other. "No. Yes. No. No. No. Yes. Yes …."

   Each of these steps is an opportunity to notice sensations in the body so that the information highway begins to open and to have a somatic experience in which each participant's yes or no is trusted and believed.

2. Shoulder Touch … Or No Shoulder Touch

   Have the participants walk around the space. If a participant would like to have their shoulder touched, they pause and another participant, if willing, will touch their shoulder. To stop the touch, the touched person can remove the hand or walk away. The touching person can also walk away. This is a non-verbal exercise that provides a somatic experience of moving in and out of touch and the act of choosing to give or receive touch. This exercise allows participants to evaluate for themselves if and when they want to give or receive touch.

3. I Want

   In this activity, participants sit in pairs and take turns saying things that they want that do not have to do with the other person.

   I want world peace.
   I want a sandwich.
   I want to go on vacation.

   Go back and forth for a couple of minutes.
   Then, switch to wants that have to do with the other participant.

   I want to touch your hair.
   I want you to tickle my ear.
   I want to sit closer to you.

The "I want you to" goes back and forth with no response to each request. This allows the participants to notice how their partner's wants make them feel. What is the somatic response? Do you feel like you have to provide the want just because it is requested? What does it feel like to ask for what you want? Can you separate the difference between "I want" and "Will you?"

Next, switch the questions to "Will you or May I." Partners go back and forth and the response to each question is always "no." This may allow partners to more easily relax into the activity because they know that the response has to be no. (It may be important to set the parameter that these are not sexual requests.)

   Will you rub my feet?
   No.
   May I touch your hair?
   No.
   Will you scratch my back?
   No.

After a few minutes of this, in the next round, allow each participant to give a genuine answer, but not execute the action. This allows them to take time, consider how they feel about the ask, and then answer genuinely with absolutely no commitment to then carry out the task. In fact, the parameter is set so that they do not complete the request.

May I sniff your ear?
No.
Will you rub my back?
Yes.
May I hold your hand.
No.

This activity encourages self noticing and reflection. Each step within the activity builds on the steps before it and includes a progression of skills used in each stage.

An Offering of Practices

The following aren't activities but are instead practices employed by teachers in higher ed that may be helpful to you in your own pedagogical work. These can all be modified to meet your individual classroom needs.

Check-In/Check-Out (Perry 2022a)

Nicole Perry, the founder of Momentum Stage, suggests allowing check-in and check-out time during class and rehearsal. This allows time for connection and is an important step in terms of building a consent-forward space. In fact, several of the activities/strategies listed in this chapter can be used as part of this check-in/check-out process. This isn't just about teacher-to-student connection, it's about student-to-student connection as well. Building connection will in turn build empathy and create a more productive learning environment. It's very easy to cram the entire class or rehearsal period with curricular/show content, but this intentional communication is equally important. Nicole explains, "I don't think check-outs happen nearly enough. We like to rehearse and teach up to the last possible second to get stuff done. Giving people time to separate from the work is important and builds community."

Red or Green (Collins Bandes 2022)

This strategy was explained to us by Patsy Collins Bandes who is the Theatre Division Chair at the Boston Conservatory at Berklee. She suggested that it works especially well in dance technique classes.

For this practice, you will need little red and green cards. It would be best if you have cards that are red on one side and green on the other. (You could even use a deck of cards with the understanding that one side represents affirmative consent and the other does not.) At the start of each class, students choose how to display the card. If they put the green card next to themselves, they are ok with physical corrections that day. The red card means no consent for physical corrections. They can revoke consent or give consent at any time during the class by flipping the card over. This practice can assist in streamlining in-class discussions: If the card is green, follow consent practices before touching (explain touch and its purpose and ask for consent to touch). If the card is red, engage with a non-touch correction.

Journaling (Kremer 2022)

Brian Kremer, associate professor of Music Theatre at Elon University suggests journaling as a strategy of communicating about productive learning environments. The journals serve as a mode of documentation for the student to report on their class experience and are then available for the teacher to read. Kremer explains that "it is not a Dear Diary … type of journal; it is more about allowing both the teacher and the students to reflect on the learning/teaching experience in order to create a productive learning space for everyone involved." We suggested earlier that it's a good idea for professors to keep journals too. They are useful to monitor progress with individual students but also function as a record of consistent pedagogy and interactions that document one-on-one time with students.

Stoplight Check-In

During our interview process, several people mentioned using this strategy which they learned as part of an Intimacy Directors and Coordinators (IDC) workshop or from others who had taken a workshop. This strategy may be used to outline individual boundaries using red, yellow, and green as categorical markers. For example, if a participant is comfortable having their left shoulder down to the left hand touched, that area would be identified as green. If the same individual is not comfortable having their hips touched by another individual, that area would be considered red. Any area that needs further discussion gets labeled as yellow. Red, yellow, and green become the framework for discussing boundaries which may be reconsidered and changed throughout the entire process.

Accessibility Check-In (Joynt Sandberg 2022b)

Before facilitating improvisational comedy practice with her students, Liz Joynt Sandberg asks them to complete an accessibility check-in with each other. This may start with body parts that may or may not be touched that day but continues into conceptual boundaries in terms of what subjects may be accessed for comedy. She explains,

> A lot of our access needs have to do with ideas and ways that we will communicate with each other. A lot of comedy is rooted and focused in language. So the accessibility check in is a great time to share if you are not available to be hugged as we are improvising together or if you do not want to infer sexual violences. This is personal for each individual. One of the ways we create community together is by advocating for ourselves.

It is also explained to the students that they may pause during the improv practice at any time if something is not working for them. The use of the pause is intentionally framed as a way to convey that something about that moment was not working and space was needed without negative connotation attached to its use.

Choice of Material (Finley 2023b)

For Rachel Finley, the choice of material is an important aspect of consent. Her own history with being assigned scenes that were not appropriate for her is at the root of her educational philosophy. She states,

> for years, many educators have taken on the approach that it is the educator who knows what material is best for the students. I choose to take the approach that each of my students know what material is best for them.

She shares with them options that are available to them, but ultimately, her students make the choices that they feel are best suited to them as individuals.

Yes/No/Maybe (Bones 2022a)

Carly DW Bones, an intimacy director, sex educator, theatre director, and community facilitator based in Los Angeles, developed this extensive form for helping actors name their personal boundaries and practice vocalizing individual needs (see Figure 8A-F). It can be used as a class exercise to help students begin thinking about boundaries or it can be adapted and used as part of an audition disclosure form for a specific show.

BOUNDARIES FOR ACTORS
YES/NO/MAYBE LIST
By Carly DW Bones

It can be easier to confidently claim your boundaries when you have a clear sense of what they are before you are in a pressured moment. Look over this list and be honest with yourself about what aligns with your needs and your integrity as an artist and a human. There are no wrong answers. What boundaries do you need to claim in order to take care of your physical, mental, emotional and spiritual health? No one else can give you your own answers.
Healthy boundaries as an actor can help you to have a sustainable career and to show up fully to do your best work. Your answers might change some over time, so do a check in a few times a year with this list as a guide. No one else needs to see this list, though you are welcome to share it with folks you are working with if that is helpful to you. You may even want to fill this out once for theatre projects and once for film projects, because your boundaries might change depending on the medium you're working in. Your answers don't need to look like anyone else's. Take what you find useful, leave what doesn't serve you, and feel free to add on.

Mark "YES" if this is something that you consent to with ease for an acting role/project.
Mark "NO" if this is a hard boundary that you do not want to do for an acting role/project.
Mark "MAYBE" if it really depends on the specifics - and elaborate in the section below!

Role that requires a full body hug/embrace	☐ YES	☐ NO	☐ MAYBE
Role that requires another actor touching my face	☐ YES	☐ NO	☐ MAYBE
Role that requires another actor touching my hair	☐ YES	☐ NO	☐ MAYBE
Role that requires kissing on the face (mouth on cheek/forehead)	☐ YES	☐ NO	☐ MAYBE
Role that requires kissing mouth on mouth	☐ YES	☐ NO	☐ MAYBE

This worksheet was created by Carly DW Bones (she/they) www.thespomancer.com

FIGURE 8A: Yes/No/Maybe worksheet created by Carly DW Bones.

Role that requires open mouth/tongue kissing	☐ YES	☐ NO	☐ MAYBE
Role that requires kissing mouth on skin (below the head)	☐ YES	☐ NO	☐ MAYBE
Role that requires me to undress on stage/film	☐ YES	☐ NO	☐ MAYBE
Role that requires me to wear see-through clothing	☐ YES	☐ NO	☐ MAYBE
Role that requires me to be in underwear/lingerie/etc.	☐ YES	☐ NO	☐ MAYBE
Role that requires me to be topless	☐ YES	☐ NO	☐ MAYBE
Role that requires me to be fully nude	☐ YES	☐ NO	☐ MAYBE
Role that requires me to change without a dressing room	☐ YES	☐ NO	☐ MAYBE
Role requiring intimacy w/out an ID/IC or intimacy trained director	☐ YES	☐ NO	☐ MAYBE
Role that requires simulated penatrative (vaginal, anal) sex	☐ YES	☐ NO	☐ MAYBE
Role that requires simulated oral (mouth) sex	☐ YES	☐ NO	☐ MAYBE
Role that requires simulated manual (hand) sex	☐ YES	☐ NO	☐ MAYBE
Role the requires simulated BDSM/Kink	☐ YES	☐ NO	☐ MAYBE
Role that requires simulated group sex	☐ YES	☐ NO	☐ MAYBE
Role that requires physical groping	☐ YES	☐ NO	☐ MAYBE
Role that requires simulated sexual violence	☐ YES	☐ NO	☐ MAYBE
Role that involves improvised physicality	☐ YES	☐ NO	☐ MAYBE
Role that stereotypes my _____ (gender, race, class, body, weight/size, sexuality, religion, disability, mental illness, profession, etc.)	☐ YES	☐ NO	☐ MAYBE
Role that contributes to stereotyping a marginalized group	☐ YES	☐ NO	☐ MAYBE
Role that stereotypes _____	☐ YES	☐ NO	☐ MAYBE

This worksheet was created by Carly DW Bones (she/they) www.thespomancer.com

FIGURE 8B: Continued.

Project where I am the only _____ in the cast (POC, woman, trans person, Black person, etc.)	☐ YES	☐ NO	☐ MAYBE
Role that explores _____ trauma (sexual, racialized, gender-based, medical, etc.)	☐ YES	☐ NO	☐ MAYBE
Role/project that asks me to access my own personal trauma	☐ YES	☐ NO	☐ MAYBE
Role that requires me to eat _____	☐ YES	☐ NO	☐ MAYBE
Role that requires me to smoke	☐ YES	☐ NO	☐ MAYBE
Role that requires me to get wet	☐ YES	☐ NO	☐ MAYBE
Role that requires me to cut or change my hair	☐ YES	☐ NO	☐ MAYBE
Role that requires me to lose weight	☐ YES	☐ NO	☐ MAYBE
Role that requires me to gain weight	☐ YES	☐ NO	☐ MAYBE
Role that requires my character to call another character a slur (racial, gendered, sexual, religious, etc.)	☐ YES	☐ NO	☐ MAYBE
Role that requires my character to be called a slur	☐ YES	☐ NO	☐ MAYBE
Role where my character speaks sexually explicit language	☐ YES	☐ NO	☐ MAYBE
Role where my character is on the receiving end of sexually explicit language	☐ YES	☐ NO	☐ MAYBE
Role where my character experiences simulated violence	☐ YES	☐ NO	☐ MAYBE
Role where my character enacts simulated violence	☐ YES	☐ NO	☐ MAYBE
Role that explores intimate partner violence	☐ YES	☐ NO	☐ MAYBE
Role that explores suicide/suicidal ideation	☐ YES	☐ NO	☐ MAYBE
Role that explores self harm	☐ YES	☐ NO	☐ MAYBE

This worksheet was created by Carly DW Bones (she/they) www.thespomancer.com

FIGURE 8C: Continued.

Role that explores disordered eating	☐ YES	☐ NO	☐ MAYBE
Role that explores death and death-related grief	☐ YES	☐ NO	☐ MAYBE
Role that requires simulated drug use	☐ YES	☐ NO	☐ MAYBE
Role/project that asks me to work for free	☐ YES	☐ NO	☐ MAYBE
Project that asks me to stay beyond the agreed time/schedule	☐ YES	☐ NO	☐ MAYBE
Project that asks me to advertise on my personal social media	☐ YES	☐ NO	☐ MAYBE
Role/project the uses my face/voice to sell _____	☐ YES	☐ NO	☐ MAYBE
Role/project that uses my face/voice to make money for _____	☐ YES	☐ NO	☐ MAYBE
Immersive show where audience can initiate touch w/ actors	☐ YES	☐ NO	☐ MAYBE
Immersive show where actors can initiate touch w/ audience	☐ YES	☐ NO	☐ MAYBE
Immersive show where alcohol is served to audience	☐ YES	☐ NO	☐ MAYBE
Immersive show that requires me to be partially/fully nude	☐ YES	☐ NO	☐ MAYBE
Immersive show where I am alone with an audience member	☐ YES	☐ NO	☐ MAYBE

ADD YOUR OWN:

_____	☐ YES	☐ NO	☐ MAYBE
_____	☐ YES	☐ NO	☐ MAYBE
_____	☐ YES	☐ NO	☐ MAYBE
_____	☐ YES	☐ NO	☐ MAYBE
_____	☐ YES	☐ NO	☐ MAYBE
_____	☐ YES	☐ NO	☐ MAYBE
_____	☐ YES	☐ NO	☐ MAYBE

This worksheet was created by Carly DW Bones (she/they) www.thespomancer.com

FIGURE 8D: Continued.

Elaborate On Your "MAYBE"s Below:

It's not unusual for many of your answers to be "MAYBE"s. What would make each "MAYBE" a clear "YES" for you? And what would make each "MAYBE" a clear "NO" for you? (Write on the back or in your journal if you need more space, and take all the space you need!)

This worksheet was created by Carly DW Bones (she/they) www.thespomancer.com

FIGURE 8E: Continued.

Practice Out Loud!

Practice saying some of these phrases out loud - to yourself, to the mirror, to a friend or roommate or fellow actor or your cat. Fill in the blanks with boundaries you have or situations you can imagine coming up. It can feel silly or cheesy at first, but saying these words out loud in a low stakes environment can help you build confidence to speak up for yourself in moments where it might be more challenging to assert your boundaries and needs. Practice helps build a kind of muscle memory that you can call upon later when there's something bigger at stake. This exercise can help you activate and realize the power of your words, and the power you wield when you tap into clear confident communication. Give it a go!

"Is _____ negotiable? I love this role but I have a hard boundary around _____ ."

"How are you planning to stage _____ ? I'd like to have some more information so I can make an informed decision before accepting this role/project."

"Will there be an intimacy choreographer/director/coordinator on board for staging _____? Or is the director specifically trained in intimacy practices? I need some more information about this before I can consent to working on this project/accept this role."

"Can you tell me a bit more about why _____ is necessary to your vision for this story?"

"Actually, _____ is a hard boundary that I have for my work. How do you think we can creatively work around it and still tell this story/realize your vision/complete this assignment?"

"While working on _____ I discovered that _____ is actually a boundary for me. How do you think we can adjust to work with respect to that discovery? Thank you so much for hearing me on this."

"I need to let you know that _____ violates a boundary that I have already communicated. If we want to continue working together, we need to address _____ . What I will need to move forward is _____. Let me know if that is doable for you so we can figure out the next steps."

"Who is the point person for me to talk to in the case that a boundary I state is being ignored or pushed? I'm not anticipating this happening, but it will make me feel safer to know in advance who I should go to directly to address this in case it comes up."

This worksheet was created by Carly DW Bones (she/they) www.thespomancer.com

FIGURE 8F: Continued.

Note: this worksheet in its entirety should not be used as is for auditions for any specific production, but rather used as a starting point that can be adapted and refined for the needs of any individual class/production. While this form is designed for actors it can be used, and adapted as needed, for any genre in the performing arts. Providing the worksheet well ahead of discussion allows time for thought and processing so that the discussion can be clearer and more productive. Sometimes we feel the pressure of time in the moment that rushes us to make decisions that are based on convenience or efficacy rather than true needs and boundaries.

Discuss Before You Measure

This strategy is costume specific, but this model of communication can be applied to any situation in performing arts education. It all boils down to the fact that information is vital. People need clear and accurate information in order to make informed decisions. Daniel Thieme-Whitlow (2022), Costume Shop Manager at Central Michigan University and Deborah Hertzberg (2022), Costume Shop Supervisor at Brooklyn College, both follow similar protocols when taking cast measurements. Preparatory information and continued conversation are the foundations of this work. Both costume professionals provide detailed information about the process, including the reason for the process, and allow for questions at any point. This happens through an initial conversation before the measurements begin. Ample time is allowed for a detailed explanation, purpose, and time for questions and modifications to the process as necessary. Then they detail and narrate each action moment by moment.

"I am now going to measure your bust" (points to own bust to indicate the body part that matches the vocabulary. Another option is to demonstrate on the dress form).

"Now I am going to do a series of measurements that go around your torso" (demonstrates on self or dress from).

Continuous check-ins allow the person being measured constant opportunities to ask questions or stop the process.

Mirroring (May 2022)

When teaching voice lessons, Joshua May, opera director at the Schwob School of Music at Columbus State University, begins class with a discussion about consent. When a student chooses not to be touched for the purpose of alignment or breath correction, he uses mirroring as a tool of instruction to achieve the same result. This method also works well for online instruction. Joshua will demonstrate what he is correcting on his own body and the student then repeats the same action on their own body. This strategy can be used in many performing arts genres and can also be used for an exercise in listening. Learning through observation keeps you rooted in the present moment and shifts the listening focus from auditory to somatic. By mirroring each other's movements, students develop skills in focus and teamwork rooted in concentration on a partner's needs and actions.

Bag of Beans (Martin 2022a)

Andrée Martin, professor of Flute in the Schwob School of Music at Columbus State University, suggests using a bag of dried beans as a tool in class for adding weight or pressure on a student's body as a corrective measure. For example, when her flute students are pulling up their shoulders, the weight from a bag of beans placed on their shoulders draws attention to that unnecessary tension and provides the somatic awareness needed to begin making the correction of releasing it. In conversations with students about consent to touch, a bag of beans is a non-touch alternative, or for some educators, Andrée included, a first-choice method. She uses this for her instrumental students, but this exercise can easily be used in a variety of performing arts disciplines. She explains, "The bag of beans doesn't carry all the information that my hand may carry." The beans are neutral. They just do the job of the corrective measure.

Modeling Apologies

Mistakes are going to happen. The work to change teaching habits is not instantaneous. Even after new habits and methods are formed, mistakes *will* continue to happen because we are human and that is part of life. You will make mistakes. Your students will make mistakes. So, let's talk about apologies. (This is also a great topic for class.) The process is not going to be perfect (there is no such thing) and modeling apologies in class will help your students be prepared to sincerely apologize when necessary and normalize this aspect of the process.

Heather's Learning (and Apology) Process

I am in the process of completely revamping my corrective teaching tools in dance. I used to touch my students all the time in order to make physical movement corrections without their permission. Now, I am implementing consent practices, but I absolutely still make mistakes. It happens. It's not easy to make this transition even though I desperately want to and believe that I am creating a better learning environment for my students. When I make a mistake I do the following:

1. I own and name my mistake without making excuses or embellishing an explanation. I am clear about what I did. "Sam, I just touched your leg to correct your stretch without asking."
2. I apologize. It is usually as simple as "I am sorry that I did that. I should have asked first."
3. I name the action that I am going to do to correct the mistake. "I will make sure to ask before making physical corrections."
4. I give the student time to respond and discuss further if needed.

I typically don't pull the student aside to apologize and I don't delay in apologizing. I apologize in the moment and right where it happened. Other students witness the apology and then this is part of creating a culture of consent and expectations that everyone will act accordingly and apologize when mistakes are made. By apologizing publicly, students see it and in turn, do the same.

Then, we also must consider the possibility that even after a sincere apology, forgiveness will not be granted. Wes Crenshaw and Greg Tangari write,

> People who are asked to receive an apology and then told they need not forgive may feel as though they're in a cultural double bind. As a society, we tend to see people who won't forgive the transgressions of others as lacking in character themselves.
>
> (Crenshaw 1998: 32)

If the classroom/rehearsal culture is created to make space for individual timing and understanding, then varying reactions to mistakes will be an acceptable and expected entity. People are all different. A uniform response to apology is unattainable if we are also grounded in honoring the human condition and its wildly varying personal responses and experiences.

An Offering of Strategies for Combating Resistance from Colleagues

This work is different from what many of us have been doing. It includes some fairly radical revisions to our teaching strategies. Therefore, it's natural for some people to resist these ideas and the changes to teaching that come with the adoption of these philosophies. So, how do we combat resistance? As Carly DW Bones reminds us, "We just want to make the best art we can and treat each other excellently while we do that. It's hard to disagree with that" (Bones 2022b). The following are ideas to include in conversations with people who are resistant to the work you are doing. Even in combating resistance though we need to remain mindful of the fact that boundaries are boundaries. Liz Joynt Sandberg reminded us that not wanting to try something new, as important as we may think it is, is in fact a boundary (Joynt Sandberg 2022c). So if we are going to do all this work to respect everyone's boundaries, then we need to do just that. We can't be intentionally selective about when we do or don't uphold the expectations. We can't ever force people to try new teaching methods, nor should we. So, these methods are conversation starters, but they aren't conversation enders, because people are in charge of themselves and the ways in which they engage with others (even when we don't like it).

Maintaining Wisdom from the Past While also Moving Forward (Bones 2022c)

Bones also suggests noting that we don't want to completely throw out all teaching and directing practices. We're not saying that everything we have done in the past is bad. There are certainly ways to maintain foundational elements of our teaching pasts while also making revisions that create healthier learning spaces for everyone involved. Bones explains,

> Our industry and our world are moving forward. Whether you choose to come with us or not, you have a ticket to get on the train to the future of making and teaching theatre. It might be a different train than you've been on before, but if you're willing to learn and grow with us then you are welcome. As we board this new train, we also don't want to lose the wisdom of our theater elders. That would be a huge disservice to the field, and there is room for both elder wisdom and new ways of caring for each other as we create together.

Power Reminder (Perry 2022b)

As educators and directors, it can be easy to forget that we hold an incredible amount of power. Nicole Perry explains,

> I think it is always a surprise to teachers when we're doing our teacher trainings and I remind them of the power dynamic that is always present in the room. They feel that because they are not major decision makers at their institution, they have no power, but that is not the case. They do hold power and it is their responsibility to learn how to hold it.

A gentle reminder about power dynamics can be a useful tool in a conversation with someone who is resistant to consent work in the classroom or rehearsal space. Students are always in a submissive position in the power dynamic and therefore are in a position to be coerced, whether unintentionally or intentionally. This work can assist in providing educators that reminder that our job is to work in a way that best serves the student, not us.

Accountability from Leadership

If consent-forward classrooms and rehearsal spaces are prioritized by leadership it will not eliminate resistance, but it may create a clearer pathway for doing this type of work. If possible, have conversations with people in leadership positions who may not necessarily be working with you in the classroom or rehearsal space, but have influence over the type of working atmosphere you want to create. Deans, chairs, artistic directors, and other people who hold institutional power are good candidates for these types of discussions.

Reinventing Is Part of It (Martin 2022b)

Andrée Martin reminded us that reinventing as a teacher is part of the process that most educators accept as they embark on the journey of being an educator. Sometimes even people who fully believe in the philosophies of consent-forward education have to be reminded of the cycle of reinvention, whether it be as a method of keeping current in one's field or a change in pedagogical strategy. Reinvention does not have to be a revolution. Small shifts and small changes in practice can be important elements of a reinvention of thinking, considering, and educating.

Student Support

For the most part, students are in favor of consent-forward learning spaces. (Actually, we have never met a student who isn't in favor of this work, but we said "for the most part," because we haven't met *all* students.) They are hungry for it. Student excitement for and investment in these processes will help spread the message. Their hunger will in itself be a motivator for some educators to begin to reflect and include some of these practices.

One Step at a Time

We can't think about this as a huge, impossible undertaking. When we allow something to overwhelm us, we tend to freeze out of fear of making a "wrong" decision rather than breaking the challenge down into manageable parts. Like any new skill, we build it one step at a time, and each step we take is better than taking no step at all.

REFERENCES

Bones, C. D. W. (2022a), interviewed by E. Daugherty and H. Trommer-Beardslee, Online 23 May 2022.

Bones, C. D. W. (2022b), interviewed by E. Daugherty and H. Trommer-Beardslee, Online 23 May 2022.

Bones, C. D. W. (2022c), interviewed by E. Daugherty and H. Trommer-Beardslee, Online 23 May 2022.

Collins Bandes, P. (2022), interviewed by E. Daugherty and H. Trommer-Beardslee, Online 23 May 2022.

Crenshaw, W. and Tangari, G. (1998), "The apology: Creating a bridge between remorse and forgiveness," *Family Therapy Networker*, 22:5, p. 32.

Finley, R. (2023a), interviewed by E. Daugherty and H. Trommer-Beardslee, Online 30 June 2023.

Finley, R. (2023b), interviewed by E. Daugherty and H. Trommer-Beardslee, Online 30 June 2023.

Hertzberg, D. (2022), interviewed by E. Daugherty and H. Trommer-Beardslee, Online 17 May 2022.

Joynt Sandberg, L. (2022a), interviewed by E. Daugherty and H. Trommer-Beardslee, Online 19 August 2022.

Joynt Sandberg, L. (2022b), interviewed by E. Daugherty and H. Trommer-Beardslee, Online 19 August 2022.

Joynt Sandberg, L. (2022c), interviewed by E. Daugherty and H. Trommer-Beardslee, Online 19 August 2022.

Kremer, B. (2022), interviewed by E. Daugherty and H. Trommer-Beardslee, Online 27 May 2022.

Martin, A. (2022a), interviewed by E. Daugherty and H. Trommer-Beardslee, Online 11 August 2022.

Martin, A. (2022b), interviewed by E. Daugherty and H. Trommer-Beardslee, Online 11 August 2022.

Martin, B. (2023), interviewed by E. Daugherty and H. Trommer-Beardslee, Online 3 July 2023.

May, J. (2022), interviewed by E. Daugherty and H. Trommer-Beardslee, Online 1 June 2022.

Pace, C. (2019), *Theatrical Intimacy Education Weekend Workshop*, Salt Lake City, UT, 2–3 November.

Pace, C. (2023), personal communication, 27 June 2023.

Pace, C. and Rikard, L. (2020a), *Staging Sex: Best Practices, Tools, and Techniques for Theatrical Intimacy*, New York, NY: Routledge, pp. 19–20.

Pace, C. and Rikard, L. (2020b), *Staging Sex: Best Practices, Tools, and Techniques for Theatrical Intimacy*, New York, NY: Routledge, p. 17.

Perry, N. (2022a), interviewed by E. Daugherty and H. Trommer-Beardslee, Online 4 May 2022.

Perry, N. (2022b), interviewed by E. Daugherty and H. Trommer-Beardslee, Online 4 May 2022.

Quinnett, K. (2022), interviewed by E. Daugherty and H. Trommer-Beardslee, Online 17 May 2022.

Rikard, L. (2022), interviewed by E. Daugherty and H. Trommer-Beardslee, Online 14 May 2022.

Steinrock, J. (2022), interviewed by E. Daugherty and H. Trommer-Beardslee, Online 29 April 2022.

Thieme-Whitlow, D. (2022), interviewed by E. Daugherty and H. Trommer-Beardslee, Central Michigan University, 20 May 2022.

6

Notes From the Field:
The Good, the Bad, and the Ugly

The following are the personal stories that we collected as we listened to practitioners share the things that have happened to them and the choices that they made along their performing and teaching journeys. Some of these stories are simply delightful. They are the stories that are beautiful in their outcomes because the participants were able to navigate tricky situations due to consent practices being in place. Some of these stories are dreadful because they were harmful in a variety of manifestations due to a lack of consent practices. Each is different and yet also grounded in the realm of similarity; they are all shared from the vantage point of learning from the past.

These stories are offered to you as sources of inspiration, empathetic companionship, and examples of what can go well and what hasn't gone well at all. We will call these instances the lessons ... some that were really hard to learn. It is our hope that this section provides information and inspiration leading to praxis within the theoretical discussions of consent-forward practices.

Methodology:
How These Stories Came to Live on These Pages

As a major portion of the research for this book, we interviewed numerous performing arts practitioners about their understanding of and experiences with consent in both education and their own performance-based journeys. Specifically, we asked,

> The book will have a notes from the field section. Can you share any specific experiences in which consent protocols, or a lack thereof, had a significant impact on a class

or rehearsal? This could be a situation where a moment could've been very tricky but because of established protocols it was more easily navigated, or a situation that you reflect on from the past that was trickier/messier/more difficult than it needed to be because these practices were not in place?

We explained that we would transcribe their stories, if they wanted to share them, and include them in the book as sources of inspiration and theoretical companionship for our readers. After the process of transcribing each story, we sent it back to each interviewee for review and asked for consent to include the story in the format that we created. Many of the storytellers made changes and some, after seeing the words on the page, asked us to delete their stories. For us, this process was theory in action and a vital component of the process that prioritized the partnership of respect and autonomy. What follows are the stories from this series of interviews.

The Bad, the Ugly, and the Super Ugly

We are going to start with the learning lessons. Yes. Every experience offers some element of a lesson, but the following stories certainly offer more opportunities for learning than some others. These are the moments, many cringe worthy, that did not go well as a result of a lack of consent-based environments.

We'll start! If we are asking people to share their stories about the stuff that didn't go well, it seems only fair that we should go first. So, here we go.

Heather's Story

About five years ago, I choreographed *The Marvelous Wonderettes*. The script calls for an audience member to be chosen as Mr. Lee, but the audience member has absolutely no idea in advance that he is to be Mr. Lee. In the story, Mr. Lee is a teacher who is the object of one of the character's, a teen girl, affection. "Mr. Lee" discovers he is Mr. Lee when the cast member sings to him and brings him onto the stage. I choreographed this song to have the cast member grab Mr. Lee's hands, sit him in a chair, touch his shoulders, and even sit on his lap. Not only did the audience member have no idea that he was going to play Mr. Lee, it happened in front of an entire audience … and we, and everyone else, thought it was hilarious. Now, knowing what I know now about consent forward performance, I am mortified, simply mortified. I am mortified for all the Mr. Lees and mortified for the cast member who did exactly what I told her to do (the choreography) with a different audience participant each night.

Elaine's Story

In my own history as an actor, there have been several experiences that would've been simpler, more comfortable, and resulted in better storytelling if time had been dedicated to the crafting of a moment of intimacy. One particular show had a character that was double cast and I had a kiss with that character. Nothing had been said about the kiss. My memory is that it didn't actually happen until the performances, but that seems wrong. Regardless, actor one and I kept it simple: lips meet, heads pivot a bit, closed mouths. Actor two had a different take on it and shoved his tongue into my mouth. Now, he was a good friend and I did not feel violated per se, but man did I feel gross in the moment. I can vividly remember the physical response I had of wanting to recoil, but needing to stay focused on the character's positive response rather than my own negative one. What's even more difficult to stomach is that I've participated in creating that same tinderbox of a situation for other actors. As a director, many years later, I asked auditioning actors to kiss because "the couple they'd be playing kiss several times in the show." Basically, show me you can do it so I won't have the work of having to create it for you. It's so gross to write about now. And, as it turns out, the all-out-go-for-it-please-cast-me kisses that happened in the audition were simply a result of the pressure of the moment and never showed up in the rehearsal room. The kisses in that show were some of the most difficult I've ever had to stage.

Keeley's Story (Stanley-Bohn 2022)

There are so many stories from my time as a professional actor in New York and Los Angeles … So many stories. These are the stories that I want to counteract. These are the stories that make me want to make the industry better for my own students.

The story that sticks with me the most is from when I was working in New York. I was in a play with a director who everyone wanted to work with. I felt honored to have this opportunity. It was a really big deal. I was playing one of the leading characters. The two main characters are in love, just discovering their love, and it was choreographed for us to touch each other's chests as we talk about the heartbeat. It was a lovely moment, but the director did not think we were getting it right. At the end of the rehearsal, the director asked me to stay …. Not the other lead actor, just me. Everyone left except for me and the director. And then he wanted to do the scene with the touching of the chests. It was just the two of us. He wasn't even in the show. I remember thinking, "You aren't my partner in this scene!" There were so many red flags. I wanted to run, but of course I stayed, because I was lucky to have *this* role with *this* director, right? It was one of those moments when the trust was just gone. Now, I want to protect my own students from these moments. That is why this work is so important.

LaToya's Story (Lain 2022)

I remember one of my male voice teachers placing his hands just below my abdominal muscles, feeling for expansion. Suddenly, his hand moved much lower than I had ever experienced from any other teacher. I remember thinking, "What do I do right now? This is uncomfortable." I just froze. I don't think he had malicious intentions, but he certainly wasn't mindful of my body's response to his touch. My body reacted to this awful moment with tension. He didn't notice. This experience was key for me as I developed as a voice teacher and how I respect my own students' boundaries. You never know what those boundaries are going to be. For some, it could be their arm. You have to ask …. And continue asking.

Jessica's Story (Steinrock 2022a)

I love improv and I love standup. In college, I was really an improv kid and after college, I continued that work professionally … But I'm a fairly petite woman who got picked up quite a bit without my consent for the sake of comedy. Sometimes I got touched in ways that did not make me feel comfortable because it was perceived to be funny. Improv is about shock, breaking patterns, and setting up an expectation and then doing the opposite. So, I was passionate about continuing to make things that are funny, but I wanted to find a way to create ethical comedy. I asked myself how we can create comedy in a space of body autonomy.

Carly's Story (Bones 2022)

There are tools, language, and frameworks that I really wish that I had earlier in my career as a director, even five years ago. If I had had these tools, I could have prevented some instances of harm between actors where I was in a position of power as a director. A lot of regret and shame can come up for me when I look back on these instances, which I think is a very human reaction to have. What's important is to not get stuck in the shame, but to do better now with the new information and knowledge that I have now. I try not to get too stuck in the past. I think humans do that to themselves a lot, especially artists. For example, one time I found out, many years later, that an actor in one of the shows I was directing held onto and acted on some character chemistry-energy toward another actor outside of rehearsal. Looking back on it now, I realize that I could have helped that situation with de-roling and defusing the chemistry between them in rehearsal—which was very charged on stage and very beautiful in the story, but should not have carried over off stage. I wish I had the tools then that I have now—I wish I had used those de-roling tools and had set up a space to encourage healthier emotional and professional boundaries between actors and also between self and character. I also learned, years later, that at callbacks for a show I directed, an actor kissed another actor on the mouth mid-scene without consent or having ever talked to them about it. I take all these lessons to heart and these days I very intentionally build spaces that are founded on consent, communication and boundaries as the path to creative collaboration.

Deb's Story (Hertzberg 2022a)

Many years ago when I was in a more junior position at a different theatre organization than my position now, I was observing a costume fitting for an actor wearing a dress that revealed the top of her breasts. The person conducting the fitting tapped the actor right on the breasts with her hands, and said "boop, boop!" (Deb's hands gesturing tapping on breasts) I couldn't believe it! We all laughed, but it was really uncomfortable and in the moment, I knew it was very inappropriate. After the actor left the woman who had touched the actor's breasts said, "I probably shouldn't have done that," and I knew she was right. I remember thinking that we needed some guidelines to protect people from that kind of behavior. You can't touch someone's body like that and as a junior employee I did not feel like I had the agency to raise the issue. It was a pretty awful feeling.

Liz's Story (Joynt-Sandberg 2022)

When I first started teaching I did not have a mentality that students are inherently capable and that it is tremendously important for their education for them to set their own agenda. I didn't understand that while I may frame out the container and the resources, the students have power. It all feels nuts to me now to look back and think about my reactions to stuff that happened. The idea that I would tell them "if you do not write this 12 page paper exactly when I want you to, something bad will happen" feels fully insane. I just remember so many feelings of being like, I am in my anger at this student and they are not respecting me and I need respect and if they don't respect me I'm going to fuck with their shit. What? What was that? I think that for me, those moments early in my time as a teacher, especially in higher education, of "how dare they" are such an indicator that I was demanding something that I was not giving. There was no mutuality in this need for respect.

The Spring Awakening *Portion of this Book*

Now we're going to talk about *Spring Awakening*. This particular show gets its own section because several people brought it up when we asked them if they could share a situation that was problematic due to a lack of having consent practices in place. Here are a few *Spring Awakening* stories.

Patsy's Story (Collins Bandes 2022a)

I was working on a professional production of *Spring Awakening* and I was the stage manager. This was a while ago. When it came time for staging the sex scene, the director wanted the actors to be completely nude …. but also didn't choreograph the intimacy for the scene. I was so uncomfortable. The actors were clearly very uncomfortable. The director said, "Just try it and see what you are comfortable with." There were other people in the room and the actors did the best they could, but they were laughing and obviously having a hard time. As the stage manager at that time, I felt like I didn't have a voice to speak up and help. Finally, the director said, "No, you are not doing it right," and sent the actors and me to another room to work it out. So, I had a long conversation with the actors and we worked out what would happen in each moment. Looking back on it now, I realize it should have never gotten to that point. It should have been something that was handled by an intimacy choreographer moment to moment and the actors should not have been completely nude. I now understand that as the stage manager, I had the authority to step up and say, "We're not doing this." In the moment though, I didn't know that I could use my voice in that way. I was complicit in how that all went down. Thankfully, we have a lot more knowledge, understanding and training now that allows us to speak up with certainty in those moments.

Tommy's Story (Wedge 2022)

When I directed *Spring Awakening,* we did not do nudity. Instead, the sex scene was staged behind a scrim. I was really focused on the ensemble choreography below them during that moment of the show. I remember telling the two actors, "I want the two of you to have a conversation about this. I'll be down here working with the ensemble, and then I'll check in with you at the end." I was totally hands-off. That's what my training was. That's how I was taught, and that's what was directed to me when I was an actor: "just go in the hall and figure it out." So what happened? The actors came up with some ideas for the scene and then I gave them my thoughts. I did feel good that I mitigated the amount of time they spent kissing as they were behind the scrim, but I later learned from one of the actors that some nights the other actor would kiss harder than other nights. This would not have happened if there had been protocols in place. Knowing what I know now, I would like to do that show again to get it right this time.

Talking with Student Actors

After hearing several references to *Spring Awakening* experiences, we decided to reach out to three actors who had previously performed the show in the roles of Wendla, Melchior, and Moritz. During our conversation, they each talked about a few uncomfortable moments in the rehearsal process for the show but mostly discussed how the lack of consent practices restricted the production's creativity. Everything was played very safely but without boundary conversations. Each of the actors reflected on the fact that if there had been a consent-forward structure in place, they could have pushed further within the storyline and created a more provocative narrative than what was actually produced (Sullivan 2022; Wilson 2022; Chu 2022).

Reflections on the Hard Lessons

Many of these stories seem to partner with regret in a way that does not value the acknowledgment of cumulative learning in relationship to the progression of time. Yet, we didn't know what we didn't know, and sometimes we still don't. We're human and growth changes our later experiences both for us and those who interact with us. Now, we have the opportunity to take these lessons and generate new methods of working that value and prioritize bodily autonomy and agency, both our students' and our own. Many of the included narratives began with unwanted or unexpected touch that resulted from an absence of having consent practices in place. Advanced planning, direct communication, and, most importantly, an innate respect as it relates to trusting other people to know what is best for themselves, is the foundation of the initial change that would have made all of these experiences better for each participant.

The Good

And now, let's jump to the good. As Ashleigh Reade stated, "These are the quieter moments. These are the moments that are sometimes harder to remember because they weren't so disruptive" (Reade 2022a).

Ashleigh's Story (Reade 2022b)

I'm thinking about a Fitzmaurice exercise that I use as part of my own teaching. I love this exercise in my own personal work and so, I offer it as an option because

I find it really useful. It's a rib massage and it gets into the intercostals. There's an option to actually pull the rib cage apart and then there's an option to do a little bit of upper abdominal massage. It's stuff that I do in practice on my own that I enjoy on my own body and so I offer it to my students with caveats. We always look at the anatomy first and then we assess the experience and the experience is always optional. I always offer a solo option and partnered work, but I have *really* crafted the solo option. It is not just an afterthought. In fact, I offer this option first. When I first started teaching, I did not have this solo option, because it was assumed that all those who entered the room were consenting to the work. Once I started offering both the solo option and the partnered work, people have been very excited, and many do both. Everyone is in control of their own experience for this exercise.

Deb's Story (Hertzberg 2022b)

So I think this was last fall. It was our first show back, first show back dealing with new COVID protocols and all of that. I had a young graduate student who did her first year online so this was the first time she was meeting us in person, and it was the first time she had a real professional costume fitting. I went through all the protocols, I asked for consent, she gave her consent, we went through the whole fitting, you know always checking in with her and providing that communication and context. At the end of the fitting, she said "Oh, thank you so much, that was really terrific. That was so easy." Then later that day she sent me an e-mail that said,

> Dear Costume Department,
> I wanted to thank you so much for your generosity and kindness in this production of *Everybody*. My first in-person show fitting was so memorable because of you all. Thank you for making my comfortability a priority. I hope to work with you again next semester.

So that just meant to me that our protocols were working because she recognized that we were prioritizing her care and comfort. And not just her comfort in her physical clothing, but her personal comfort in the fitting environment. And it gave me so much more motivation for continuing this work because I knew that it was concretely working.

Heather's Story

I was teaching a swing dance class recently and I realized that if I was really committed to this work, I would have to give a non-touch option—and not just as a "less than" option. I introduced the class by offering two options. One option was with traditional hand held touch. The other was partner work that relied on connection without touching. Really, rhythm is the contract in swing anyway. There was absolutely no difference in success between the touchers and the non-touchers. Everyone rocked around the room. The music was loud and it was super sweaty. And everyone was cool with it. People who wanted to touch did. People who did not want to touch didn't. It was fun and a lot of learning about partner work happened that day.

Patsy's Story (Collins Bandes 2022b)

One of our seniors this past year wanted to direct the play *Mediocre Heterosexual Sex*. I remember thinking, "What are you talking about!?" I read it and there was some obvious physical intimate contact on stage. Again, I thought, "How are we possibly going to do this?!" I was trying really hard to not just say, "Nope," and be done with it. The student was passionate about the project and so we asked them to work with a faculty member step by step through the play to develop procedures .... And they did. They worked to create plans using shields, appropriate undergarments, and positioning. They did the entire play without any nudity and outlined every moment as part of their rehearsal plan. This included consent protocols and modifications depending on boundaries and other factors. It ended up that this student could engage actively with this piece of material that really spoke to them in a new and creative way. I definitely learned from this process and I am glad we did not say no without giving the student an opportunity to work through the planning process that became part of the proposal to the faculty. The moment we said yes to the proposal felt celebratory!

Chels's Story (Morgan 2022)

Last year I wrote and directed a short film called *Let Them Be Loved*. On the day of shooting, one of the worst things that can happen to a director happened—an actor dropped out about thirty minutes before call. It was for COVID-related reasons, so completely understandable, but it still left me trying to figure out what to do. Everything we had rehearsed and created was gone. It was a film about two queer men and there was so much wrapped up in this important project with many professionals involved. I had to figure out what to do. It was intimidating. But there were many intimacy coordinators involved in the project and I used those resources—those ideas—as a guide. We asked a lot of questions. We talked. As we were getting ready to shoot, I rebuilt and rechoreographed with another actor who happened to be on set as a member of the crew. Denise Khumalo, an intimacy coordinator from Intimacy Coordinators of Color, and I were able to work with the actors to establish their new boundaries and they trusted us. They trusted us because we were doing the work and asking a lot of questions. We were all flexible and we all trusted the process because we talked through the entire thing and we had already established a framework of consent that the new actor was able to find a place within. We had already created an environment of trust. Everyone knew that their boundaries would be respected and that is one of the biggest takeaways from this work. This business requires a lot of creativity. You have to be ready to make a plan B and even a plan C. There are many ways to tell a story.

Jessica's Story (Steinrock 2022b)

I was working as the intimacy director for a production and we were working on a romantic scene in which one character (played by "Actor A") needed to jump into the arms of another character (played by "Actor B"). We had consent protocols in place and we discussed boundaries for this embrace. The "Actor A" identified the boundary that they did not want their rear to be touched. As a group, we worked on choreographing the scene in such a way that respected that boundary. "Actor B" was able to lift them up in a way that worked for the scene and respected the boundaries that had been set. However, during a rehearsal when "Actor A" jumped into their partner's arms it did not go as planned. "Actor B" wasn't able to stabilize and accidentally came in contact with "Actor A's" backside, crossing the established boundary. We stopped immediately. "Actor B" apologized and explained what happened. The two actors had already built up trust with each other which allowed for quick repair. We realized that the jump into the embrace was not going to be able to be consistent in terms of the set boundary, so we adjusted the choreography. Using a scoop motion rather than a jump would give "Actor B" more control. It looked great, respected the set boundary, and still told the story that we needed to tell. There was an apology, repair, and then immediate action to protect that boundary.

Joshua's Story (May 2022)

(Authors' note: This story is going to start off sounding like a lesson learned, but hold tight. This is definitely a success story and, honestly, a situation that many performers will find themselves in. This type of situation is worth talking about with our students. Sometimes there won't be consent practices in place, absolutely not ideal, but as they encounter these moments they can advocate for themselves and their scene partners in the manner described by Joshua.)

Back to Joshua's Story

I remember a time when I was in a show and we were working on an intimate scene on a bed. The instructions from the director were. "Just go for it. Experiment and see how it goes." I felt so uncomfortable in that moment. I stopped and took a moment to discuss boundaries with my scene partner. We talked about our comfort level, personal boundaries, and ideas for the scene. We planned what we were going to try and if something didn't work, we discussed it and came up with a solution that worked for both of us. This created a good situation out of something that could have been really awful. We had five minutes that we needed to fill on the bed. That is an eternity! There is no way that either of us would have felt comfortable "just going for it."

Sarah's Story (Lozoff 2022)

One of my most recent productions in which I was the intimacy director for the show, went so smoothly, I felt like maybe I wasn't needed. I completely second-guessed myself. But I was needed, that is the thing about this kind of work. I think of it this way … I was the person there for when everyone else wanted to light stuff on fire and I would talk with them about how to protect the stuff that they did not want to light on fire. I was the person standing in the corner with a fire extinguisher. One of the most difficult things that I found was convincing everyone involved in making the show that while there were moments that felt like compromising, we really just had to be open enough to explore what other options there were. I firmly believed that we were not going to end up feeling like we were settling for compromise, but we could find a better option for everyone across the board. It was an interesting process for me because it was not actually staging any kind of simulated intimacy. It was in the broader part of advocacy and facilitating healthy communication and it went really well. The same is true when I work with professional dance companies. In professional dance, it's still not standard for there to be a stage manager in the room. That's really different from theatre and I think ultimately unfair to the choreographer at the front of the room because they also have to wear that hat in terms of keeping track of the time and breaks and everything else in terms of taking care of the dancers. My work with dancers is around consent. It's around advocacy. It's around healthy communication.

Zev's Story (Steinrock 2022c)

Recently, in a stage combat class that I was teaching, I had a student call stop as we were working on an exercise with swords. They said, "I actually do not want to be touched today." They felt confident enough to say this in the moment. It was so succinct and so immediate. There was something about the atmosphere that we had built together as a community that gave them confidence and allowed them to exert their power. I thanked them and congratulated them on asking for what they needed. There's such a huge pressure in the performing arts for performers and students to not be difficult and there is this idea that having needs makes you difficult. After many years of not doing so, I am now working to actively and consistently remind my students to ask for what they need. And when they do this, I believe it is very important to congratulate them.

Reflections on the Good Moments

It is interesting to note that most of these good moments are fairly recent in relationship with the timing of the interviews; they aren't stories from the distant past. We think this has less to do with a distinction between methods of working over time, although this could also be significant in some cases, and more to do with the disruptive nature of these experiences. That disruption has made them more memorable over the course of time. The good moments can sometimes fade because they are not disruptive, but rather integrate smoothly into the experience without significant reflection, and therefore simply exist without conscious note. Each of the stories resulted from a moment of acknowledgment that an additional step was needed to care for the involved participants. Whether structural or improvised due to an immediate need, that additional step grounded each of these experiences in a valuing of human empathy.

REFERENCES

Bones, C. D. W. (2022), interviewed by E. Daugherty and H. Trommer-Beardslee, Online 23 May 2022.

Chu, B. (2022), interviewed by E. Daugherty and H. Trommer-Beardslee, Online 13 June 2022.

Collins Bandes, P. (2022a), interviewed by E. Daugherty and H. Trommer-Beardslee, Online 23 May 2022.

Collins Bandes, P. (2022b), interviewed by E. Daugherty and H. Trommer-Beardslee, Online 23 May 2022.

Hertzberg, D. (2022a), interviewed by E. Daugherty and H. Trommer-Beardslee, Online 17 May 2022.

Hertzberg, D. (2022b), interviewed by E. Daugherty and H. Trommer-Beardslee, Online 17 May 2022.

Joynt-Sandberg, L. (2022), interviewed by E. Daugherty and H. Trommer-Beardslee, Online 19 August 2022.

Lain, L. (2022), interviewed by E. Daugherty and H. Trommer-Beardslee, Online 14 June 2022.

Lozoff, S. (2022), interviewed by E. Daugherty and H. Trommer-Beardslee, Online 1 June 2022.

May, J. (2022), interviewed by E. Daugherty and H. Trommer-Beardslee, Online 1 June 2022.

Morgan, C. (2022), interviewed by E. Daugherty and H. Trommer-Beardslee, Online 31 May 2022.

Stanley-Bohn, K. (2022), interviewed by E. Daugherty and H. Trommer-Beardslee, Central Michigan University, 10 June 2022.

Steinrock, J. (2022a), interviewed by E. Daugherty and H. Trommer-Beardslee, Online 29 April 2022.

Steinrock, J. (2022b), interviewed by E. Daugherty and H. Trommer-Beardslee, Online 29 April 2022.

Steinrock, Z. (2022c), interviewed by E. Daugherty and H. Trommer-Beardslee, Online 26 May 2022.

Sullivan, C. F. (2022), interviewed by E. Daugherty and H. Trommer-Beardslee, Online 13 June 2022.

Reade, A. (2022a), interviewed by E. Daugherty and H. Trommer-Beardslee, Online 31 May 2022.

Reade, A. (2022b), interviewed by E. Daugherty and H. Trommer-Beardslee, Online 31 May 2022.

Wedge, T. (2022), interviewed by E. Daugherty and H. Trommer-Beardslee, Online 25 May 2022.

Wilson, S. (2022), interviewed by E. Daugherty and H. Trommer-Beardslee, Online 13 June 2022.

Conclusion

Consent-forward classrooms are simple in their philosophical groundings in human respect and yet sometimes seemingly complex in their execution as they relate to the intricacies of human emotional subtext. This stuff can be exciting and overwhelming all at the same time. But once you see it, you can't unsee it.

Actively engaging in consent-forward practices can assist in easing the power hierarchies in our educational spaces, and one of the fastest ways to begin implementing these practices is to develop the new habit of asking before touching. Tell the student what you aim to do and why and give them the opportunity to permit or deny this action. Want to assist your dancer with their extension? Want to help your clarinetist adjust their hand positioning? Want your vocalist to shift their posture for improved breath support? Ask before you reach for them. Wait for their answer. Move forward in a manner that honors the response.

In addition, the following is offered to you as you continue on this journey.

Highlights Reel

1. Consent is not just about yes and no. Consent requires continuous communication and active engagement from all participants.
2. It is impossible to fully eliminate the hierarchical power dynamic in the classroom, but we can take steps as educators to mitigate it.
3. Students have power. What we need to ask ourselves as educators is, "How are we going to engage in the classroom so that students have the agency to use their power?"
4. Students have boundaries. (So do teachers!) It is necessary to create classroom and rehearsal spaces that provide space for everyone to articulate those boundaries and remain autonomous.
5. The development of a programmatic policy can set the tone for consistent consent-based practices in an organization. Community creation of the policy will increase stakeholder investment.

Quick Tips for Creating Consent Forward Classrooms

1. Be willing to objectively assess how you work and make changes as needed.
2. You don't have to implement all your ideas at once. Try one thing and implement that. If it works, great. If it doesn't, modify it until it does.
3. Decide on the idea that seems most manageable to you and implement that first. Community Agreement? Discussing boundaries with students? No touch/low touch/permission to touch correction methods?
4. Keep going back to the idea of autonomy. Are your classroom practices prioritizing and encouraging student autonomy?
5. Ask your students open-ended questions and be prepared to not get the answer you want. Respect their response and have equitable, alternate options available.
6. Normalize saying no. No can be really hard. The word option means that there are choices, but if yes is the only "option" that's not actually a choice.
7. Let your students know you are re-examining your teaching practices. Be honest about it.
8. Reach out! You do not have to do this work alone. You are not expected to have all the ideas all the time. Find someone to brainstorm with you. Talk through ideas, strategies, modifications, failures, and successes.
9. Consent practices are varied and not one-size-fits-all. Adapt these offerings and make the changes that fit your classroom needs.

An Important Reminder About Mistakes

You are going to make them. We're going to say that again with emphasis. **You are going to make mistakes.** This is not a perfect process and you are a human taking risks. Humans taking risks make mistakes. It may be helpful to your process if you just go ahead and give yourself permission to make mistakes right now so you are not shocked when you inevitably make them later. Take accountability and do the work ... if you want to, of course. It's always your choice.

What's Next?

Many of the people we talked with in the process of researching this book discussed their next steps in creating consent-forward classrooms and rehearsal spaces. These plans ranged from continuing to contemplate consent-forward ideas to writing books about consent practices. Many people discussed collaborating with their departments or groups of teaching partners to implement some of these ideas throughout their entire program. What's your next step? (Seriously, we want to know. Please write to us and let us know what you are doing … we may want to try it in our own classrooms.)

About the Authors

Elaine DiFalco Daugherty (she/her), MFA, MA, is an assistant professor in the Department of Theatre and Dance at Central Michigan University. She has led intimacy and consent sessions for the American Association of Community Theatre, Community Theatre Association of Michigan, KCACTF, MI Thespian Festival, University of Idaho, Casper College Wyoming, Millersville University, and has introduced consent practices to theatre, dance, costume, and sound classes. Her play, *Watermelon in Wartime*, was featured in the 2022 Voices of Truth Festival at Powerstories Theatre and earned her an Author Fellowship to The Martha's Vineyard Institute of Creative Writing. She has published articles in *Theatre Topics* and *Journal of Applied Arts and Health*.

Heather Trommer-Beardslee (she/her), MFA, MA, is the coordinator of the Central Michigan University Dance Program and artistic director of the University Theatre Dance Company. Her concert dances and dance films have been performed/screened nationally and internationally and her articles have been published in the *Journal of Dance Education*, *Teaching Artist Journal*, *Journal of Applied Arts and Health*, and *Dance Education in Practice*. Her book project, *Removing the Educational Silos: Models of Interdisciplinary and Multidisciplinary Education* was released in Fall 2022 (Intellect). For ten years, she worked for the Emmy-Award winning, Chicago-based dance company, Jump Rhythm Jazz Project as their booking manager and executive director. Heather used many of these experiences and her work as a manager and teacher at two dance studios in writing her textbook, *Dance Production and Management* (Princeton Book Company, 2013).

Index

www.ingramcontent.com/pod-product-compliance
Ingram Content Group UK Ltd.
Pitfield, Milton Keynes, MK11 3LW, UK
UKHW051007311224
453005UK00004B/19